Childless: no choice

What does involuntary childlessness mean to those people who suffer from it and how can they be helped?

As many as one in five couples in some population groups might be involuntarily childless and, despite the attention attracted by technological advances and media coverage, people often feel themselves to be totally isolated, stigmatised, and misunderstood by many professionals and ordinary people. *Childess: No Choice* is based on original research into the emotional and social aspects of involuntary childlessness, the main component being a long-term study of the experiences of couples attending a fertility clinic, supported by a community survey and a study of the attitudes of general practitioners.

At a time of rapidly developing treatments for infertility and new legislative controls, it is important that all those professionally involved have a full appreciation of the experiences and views of infertile people themselves. While there is enormous attention in the media given to getting pregnant and to childbirth, there is an almost total neglect of the possibility that for some people these 'natural' functions may not happen. James H. Monach examines in detail the impact of childlessness and the availability of choices for childless people including artificial insemination, fostering and adoption.

This book will be invaluable to doctors, sociologists, social workers, psychologists, health administrators and to anyone who works with childless couples, as well as to childless couples themselves.

James H. Monach is a Senior Lecturer in Social Work at Sheffield Hallam University.

Childless: no choice

The experience of involuntary childlessness

James H. Monach

London and New York

First published in 1993
by Routledge
11 New Fetter Lane, London EC4P 4EE

Simultaneously published in the USA and Canada
by Routledge
29 West 35th Street, New York, NY 10001

© 1993 James H. Monach

Typeset in Times by LaserScript Limited, Mitcham, Surrey
Printed and bound in Great Britain by
TJ Press (Padstow) Ltd, Padstow, Cornwall

British Library Cataloguing-in-Publication Data

A catalogue record for this book is available from the British Library.

Library of Congress Cataloging-in-Publication Data

Monach, James H., 1948-
Childless: no choice: the experience of involuntary childlessness/by James H.
  Monach.
    p. cm.
  Includes bibliographical references and index.
    1. Childlessness – England – Psychological aspects – Case studies.   2.
Infertility – England – Psychological aspects – Case studies.   I. Title.
HQ616.M66   1993
 306.87–dc20
                                                          92-26075
                                                              CIP

ISBN 0-415-04090-6

To Jane, also my Father, Kate, Jenni and John for all their love, patience and encouragement

Contents

List of tables and figure

Acknowledgements

In an enterprise of this size, covering ten years, the list of those to whom one becomes indebted grows very long. The main debt is owed to my wife, Jane, without whose support, personal sacrifice and constant encouragement the project would long since have ended. The rest of my family have provided unstinting support in all sorts of ways. My mother and my father brought me up to value knowledge and my father, John Monach, has housed me whilst writing, coded data and proof read with endless care and patience.

Professor Cooke gave advice and access to the Infertility Clinic; Professor Eric Sainsbury and David Phillips of the University of Sheffield, the academic supervisors of the research upon which this book is based, gave invaluable support and guidance. The research would not have been completed without them. The following people have also played an important part in the compilation of this book: Dr Simon Barley, Dr Jeanette McGorrigan, Dr Stephen Wright and Mary Kerrigan with the General Practice Survey; Dr Lawrence Kershaw and the staff of the Sheffield Family Health Services Authority with the Family Practitioner Survey; the Nuffield Foundation, the National Association for the Childless, Sheffield Grammar Schools Fund, Sheffield City Polytechnic, Richardson Merrell Ltd, and Derbyshire County Council for financial and practical assistance; the staff of the University of Sheffield Computing Services, especially Roger Richards, and the Sheffield City Polytechnic Computer Services; Joan Taylor and Trudi Parsons for secretarial support; Chris Lyons and staff, Trent Regional Health Authority, for computer coding. In addition, I am glad to record my thanks to colleagues at Sheffield City Polytechnic for their support, in particular Martin King.

My sincere thanks are due especially to the respondents to these surveys: Sheffield GPs, the patients of Dr Barley's practice and, above all, the patients of Professor Cooke, who gave generously of their time and emotional energy. Their answers to my questions about their experiences, frequently painful to recall, comprise the real substance of this study. Finally, I am pleased to record my thanks to Routledge and also to Heather Gibson for her patience and confidence.

1 Childless: the context

Childlessness is regarded in many different ways in our society, at best as a misfortune, at worst as irresponsibility or deviance.

With the advent of reliable contraception and worldwide concern about over-population it has now been accepted that small families are 'socially responsible', but not, still, 'no family' (the everyday shorthand for 'no children', which childless people find demeaning). Voluntary childlessness has still to gain wholehearted social approval, and is often acknowledged as indicative of covert disability. Involuntary childlessness is, statistically at least, a deviant family form, and one which has attracted little open concern and interest. Until recently, very little attention has been paid to the situation of those couples who wish to have children, but fail to conceive. Medical intervention might help, but this might be very demanding, and, in many cases, ultimately unsuccessful.

At the time that this study was proposed, there was very little in the literature of the social sciences that dealt directly with this matter, other than to the extent that it impinged on the provision of adoption services. Humphrey wondered 'why childlessness has been a theme for the creative artist rather than for the social scientist' (Humphrey 1969: 130). The question is still relevant. The available, factual literature was concentrated in the medical field: the concerns of social science emerged, almost exclusively, in the consideration of the possibility of there being a substantial psychological component in the etiology of infertility.

The concerns of social work, in particular, appeared to have been solely those of the adoption services. The interest in social work service to the infertile couple themselves, for that reason, had been very little indeed, other than in support of those investigating the hypothesised psychogenesis of infertility, or in treating those for whom no explanation of their infertility could be found. Counselling for the infertile had barely been identified as a need, other than as a very small part of the interests of the medical social work service.

This book is based on a research project conceived during a period in which I was responsible for the provision of a fostering service in a county social services department. It was clear that such a service, perhaps necessarily, could only perceive childless couples as a resource for children requiring substitute family care. It was not geared to responding to the pain such couples were experiencing in their failure to conceive a child. It was getting very difficult for such couples to find an adoption agency willing to accept them, even on to a waiting list. Many agencies had closed waiting lists some years before, and were needing to recruit only a very limited number of new adoptive parents each year, in view of the dramatic fall in the number of new-born babies requiring adoption.

This appeared to have several effects on the situation faced by the fostering service. Firstly, some of these couples were motivated primarily by the need for a child in their family. This was unlikely to be compatible with the demands placed on foster parents to share care, often temporarily, with both natural parents and the local authority. Many of these couples came with a burden of anger and pain at their failure to conceive as simply and as naturally as so many others seemed to be doing in society. The anger they felt was often compounded by their experiences of medical services, which many perceived as impersonal and insensitive to their needs and feelings. This was exacerbated when they were advised to seek adoption as their only realistic hope of obtaining a child, only to be met by social services who appeared unable to meet their needs, who indeed frequently made it plain that they saw, as their first priority, the children in their care, and potential adopters as an abundant resource. Because of the abundance of would-be adopters, agencies had made increasingly restrictive regulations about those people who would be considered for vetting and, it was felt, had become even more restrictive in the unpublished criteria applied to the vetting process.

Personal experience suggested that the anger and pain referred to above was far from resolved at the time that would-be adopters or foster parents contacted the social services. In many cases, it seemed that the first requirement of the social work service was to offer this opportunity of resolution to the couple concerned, that is, the chance, in a non-threatening and non-judgemental way, to look at these feelings and experiences, gaining some control over them in the process. This would enable other parenting tasks to be considered, less clouded by the emotional consequences of their failure to conceive. The feeling frequently expressed was that of being on a treadmill, which moved at a predetermined pace geared to its own needs. To get off this treadmill would spell the end of the couple's hopes. The factor of age was felt to be particularly important, in view of the widespread use of age limits. This was perceived as a thinly disguised form of rationing in the adoption service, as agencies made little effort to justify the hypothes-ised adverse effects of a substantial age gap between parents and child.

Couples also often expressed, in verbal or non-verbal ways, the 'double bind' they felt placed in with regard to these unresolved feelings. In their view, possibly directly confirmed by social services, the existence of these painful feelings was regarded as inevitable by the social worker, but also as being a disqualifying factor against their acceptance in one of these sub-stitute parenting roles. They felt that 'the system' required them to be frank and open about these feelings, but was likely to discriminate against them if they were too frank.

Both personal and professional contact with involuntarily childless people emphasised the extent to which they felt 'outsiders', 'odd', 'differ-ent' when compared to their contemporaries – comparisons which they felt were being made all the time. They seemed to 'see themselves as different from and, therefore, less good than their child-bearing friends and relatives and less good than their own parents who conceived and bore them' (Barry 1961: 51–2). Linked to this was the extent to which, for these couples and the 'significant others' whom they felt adding to the pressure, having a child was regarded as the natural and inevitable consequence of marriage (as distinct from a settled, heterosexual relationship). The question asked about family intentions of the wife was always 'when', not 'why' or 'if'. These pressures will be discussed later as pronatalism.

Childlessness has received scant attention from social work or the wider social sciences. No previous systematic attempt had been made to evaluate the experiences of infertile people in relation to their failure to conceive a child, and in relation to the services to which they are exposed in the course of the investigation of their infertility. The literature in fiction and in personal accounts served to emphasise the extent of the personal pain experienced, and thus to point up the need for a careful study of these experiences.

On a wider level, it was noted that there was no British epidemiological evidence, regarding the incidence of subfertility in the community, against which to compare the take up of medical service. At a very early stage, it appeared that those involved in the provision of specialist medical services felt that there was a clear socio-demographic bias in the population of referrals towards the better educated and higher income groups. There was no evidence that they were any more likely to suffer impaired fertility than other groups in the population. The only epidemiological evidence on this point, published in the United States since the completion of this research, suggests a correlation in the opposite direction; infertile women and their husbands were significantly less likely to have higher status jobs than those with children (Hirsch and Mosher 1987).

This book will address these issues: the extent of the problem of infertility and the impact it has on both the individual and the couple affected.

TERMINOLOGY

There is some confusion in the way important terms are used in this field, which merits a note of explanation. 'Sociological' is used here in a general, not technical, sense.

Infertility   Widely used in the sociological and medical literature to connote the failure of a woman to achieve pregnancy or carry a child to term, or of a man to cause pregnancy. In medical practice, a commonly used clarification is that this failure should be of at least one year's duration of regular, unprotected sexual intercourse.

Subfertility   Sometimes in medical usage, where there is a known or demonstrable impairment of reproductive capacity which falls short of total sterility.

Fertility   (1) In medical or sociological usage, the reproductive capacity, proved or otherwise, of a man or woman. (2) In demography, achieved reproductive capacity with reference to individuals and populations.

Fecundity   In demography and some sociological usage, the counterpart of fertility; that is the innate capacity or potential to reproduce or procreate.

Subfecundity   As fecundity, in cases of impaired capacity or potential to reproduce or procreate.

Sterility   The, usually irreversible, inability of an individual to reproduce; normally used only in relation to demonstrable pathology.

Childless   (1) Without children born to that individual or the individual's partner; normally subclassified as voluntary or involuntary; the term 'intentional' is sometimes used synonymously with 'voluntary' (e.g. Baum and Cope 1980). (2) Occasionally used as meaning childless by choice.

Childfree   Having chosen not to have children, as a conscious decision.

Parous   Women who have conceived and given birth to a child.

Childedness   The status of women in relation to having or not having had children.

In the course of this book the terms used, unless otherwise stated, will be: 'infertility' in the sense given above; 'fertility' in sense (1) above, i.e. *not* the demographic sense; 'childless' in the involuntary sense, i.e. sense (1); other terms, without alternative senses described, to be used as given above.

The expressions 'involuntary' and 'voluntary' misleadingly suggest that there is a clear boundary between those who choose not to have children and those who do not have the choice. However, the work done on voluntary childlessness in North America (e.g. Veevers 1979, Houseknecht 1979) and in Britain (e.g. Baum 1980, Porter 1980) and this study of involuntary childlessness, confirm what has been suspected, that the boundary may shift. There are those who enter marriage, or long-term heterosexual relationships, with the intention of having children, whilst others intend not to have children. There are also those who intend having children, but who later discover a fertility problem, and are unsuccessful. This latter group may subsequently define their condition as being child-free: they came to see the advantages of life without parenthood, and perhaps chose not to take all the steps available to them to resolve the childlessness, either medically or 'socially' (by adoption, etc.). As the decision to 'try' for children is delayed, the sums may change. Similarly, those who did not intend to have children initially, and thus considered themselves to be childfree, may subsequently decide to try for children, yet find themselves infertile.

It is probably more helpful to consider childlessness in general as a continuum, on which there are those clearly at either end, but there is a group in the middle whose position is not so simple and might change over time.

NATURE OF THE RESEARCH

Overall, the aims were to improve our understanding of the personal meanings of infertility and its impact on the individuals affected and their relationships, and of those factors which govern the decision to identify childlessness as a problem which requires medical intervention. Out of this better understanding, it is hoped that the study will contribute to debate concerning the proper design of medical and social service facilities offered to the childless as treatment and as alternative parenting opportunities. It is hoped that this will balance and inform the development of services at a time of great medical advances in treatment, which could have the effect of exacerbating the stress experienced by the couples under investigation.

There were three key elements in the research described in this book. Full descriptions and discussions, as well as copies of the research instruments themselves, can be found in the thesis which first presented this research (Monach 1987).

Infertility clinic survey

Thirty couples were recruited from new referrals to a specialist infertility clinic, to take part in this longitudinal study. This Clinic took place weekly at the instigation of a university department of obstetrics and gynaecology, in a National Health Service hospital for women. The Clinic was not formally funded at the time, but received most of the local referrals for specialist investigation. The consultant responsible saw some patients (the more apparently straightforward, or of particular research interest) in his research clinic, and the rest in this Infertility Clinic.

The couples invited to participate in the research, which was clearly explained at the outset, had not previously conceived a child *in that relationship*, nor had specialist investigation. The couples were interviewed three times over a period of four-and-a-half years.

Intake interview

This interview, which lasted approximately 30 to 40 minutes, took place in a private office in the Clinic immediately following the first medical consultation, or at home shortly afterwards if both partners were not present at the Clinic. The couples were first asked about their personal circumstances, history of their relationship, the history of their attempts to become parents, and then asked to rate themselves and their partners on a range of scales about their feelings and personalities (this questionnaire was swapped for 'marking', i.e. agreement or disagreement by the other partner after completion).

First follow-up

This occurred approximately six months after intake, by which time the basic tests were completed and the general nature of the problem had been identified, but the more intensive treatments (if indicated by tests) had not yet begun. In all but one case, they were conducted at the respondents' own home, and lasted between 60 and 90 minutes. The respondents were asked about social activities, experiences of infertility and the investigation process.

Second follow-up interview

The final interview, conducted in the respondents' own home, took place about four years after the second interview, by which time the majority had reached a 'resolution' of their childlessness whether through pregnancy or acceptance of remaining childless. This interview could last up to four hours. They were asked once again to rate themselves and their partners on scales used in the first interview, their feelings about the infertility and its investigation, and any alternative strategies they had explored (e.g. donor insemination, adoption), their views on the impact of infertility on them and their relationships, and the patterns of organisation in their relationship and social network.

During the period of the research the rapid expansion of treatment possibilities meant that some couples were still in treatment, or on waiting lists for treatment, after four-and-a-half years. This period coincided with the early phase of the development of the reproductive technologies which have flowed from the pioneering of *in vitro* fertilisation methods by Steptoe and Edwards (Winston 1986). There can be no entirely satisfactory cut-off point for such a research project as some couples known to this clinic had persisted for 12 years and more in their pursuit of a successful pregnancy; indeed the continuous introduction of scientific advances in treatment guarantees that some couples may persevere for as long as a treatment service is willing to offer hope.

The couples who joined the research gave permission to have their medical files accessed, and in return received a guarantee of absolute confidentiality for their information. Personal details are altered and names are changed to protect their identities in this book. The interviews were all conducted by the author, and recorded by handwritten notes, but verbatim where possibly significant responses were involved. The interviews used both structured and semi-structured questionnaires.

All interviews were of the husband and wife together to maximise the information available of their shared and individual perceptions; given the focus on the relationship it was felt that separate interviews might only exacerbate the stress experienced by the couples. The only exceptions were later interviews with the two couples whose marriages broke up during this period. With one exception the couples were all legally married, and as the exception was publicly presented as a marriage, the titles 'husband' and 'wife' will be used throughout as an accurate reflection of the usage of all the couples. The experience of those women wishing to have children without a heterosexual partner or in less formal co-habitations will in many ways be similar; however, they were not represented in this study. Given the attitudes discussed later, it is not surprising that such women are not found in infertility clinics in larger numbers.

All the couples initially recruited remained in the study throughout the period, with the exception of two women, one who separated from her husband early in this period, and another who refused to take part in the final interview.

It was recognised that referrals to this service might not be representative of the population at large. Townsend and Davidson (1982) suggest that specialist hospital services, other than accident and emergency clinics, are under-used by the lower socio-economic groups in our community. In preparatory discussions for this study, a doctor observed that the patient population of the Infertility Clinic tended to be 'middle class, professional, atypical of the area as a whole, and quite a determined and anxious group as well'. The study confirmed that referrals were not representative of the area, although not quite in this way. The study group did prove to be representative of referrals as a whole.

General practice survey (GPS)

In order to obtain information on infertility in the community, particularly amongst those groups who might be under-represented in a specialist clinic, a general practice survey was undertaken.

A group general medical practice, with an established research interest, based on a deprived, working-class public housing estate, agreed to co-operate with a questionnaire survey of their patients. As is discussed in the next chapter, there is little sound epidemiological evidence as to the true extent of infertility experienced in the general population. This survey represents, at the least, an attempt to sketch in the outlines of the problem.

The area chosen was felt to be appropriate not just for the pragmatic (and by no means insignificant) reason that the doctors supported the aims of the research, but also because of the characteristics of the population that they served. A deprived urban estate might be expected to have a lower take-up of specialist infertility services. In addition the working-class patients referred would least closely fit the widespread stereotype of the socio-economic characteristics of infertility clinic attenders. The practice doctors were already interested in the possibility of a questionnaire survey of some kind to establish a consistent baseline, in all medical notes, of information about key personal, social, and medical circumstances. Fertility would be a necessary part of these data.

A postal questionnaire was devised, in co-operation with the doctors, which would meet both requirements. That is a socio-medical history from which it would be possible to identify those who might have fertility problems which could be further investigated with a follow-up questionnaire. The initial questionnaire, designed in accordance with proven methodologies, was piloted in another practice in the same city, and appropriate adjustments made. All patients over the age of 18 in the practice, 3,948 in all, had a personal copy of the questionnaire delivered to their home address with a stamped, addressed return envelope. A total of 2,388 (60.5 per cent) returned this questionnaire. Unfortunately about a dozen of the patients complained at being asked to complete it, which caused the doctors to withdraw their agreement to a reminder being sent out to those who had not returned the form. The response rate is, therefore, a good one in the circumstances. (A similar study in Canada produced a response rate of just 68 per cent with the advantage of two reminders (Siemiaticki *et al.* 1984).) As the practice is geographically concentrated, it was possible to compare the respondents with the local population on a number of the parameters covered by the Census 1981 (OPCS 1981a). It was found that the survey group closely mirrored the community in respect of their sex distribution, place of birth, marital status, and the proportion of child-bearing age.

It was possible to identify three groups of women amongst those who responded, distinguished according to whether or not they were living in a heterosexual partnership during their fertile years, using contraception (including sterilisation), and cited difficulties in having children:

1 *childless* – exposed to the possibility of pregnancy, yet has not given birth to a live child;
2 *childfree* – exposed to the possibility of pregnancy but delaying or avoiding childbirth by contraception or sterilisation;
3 *parous* – with one or more previous, successful pregnancies.

The difficulties of any categorisation of this kind are further discussed in Chapter 2. In the study 222 women were identified as falling into groups 1 and 2. Excluding those over the age of 45, who it was felt might find enquiries about their fertility less acceptable, 51 women falling into groups 1 and 2 were approached to complete a second questionnaire which directly addressed issues of fertility and parenting intentions.

Family practitioner survey (FPS)

In the course of this research, the role of the general practitioner (GP) was discussed with the clinic patients. It became apparent that the GP was felt to have been a very significant figure for many of the couples concerned, for both good *and* ill, at least at some stages of the investigation and treatment. An opportunity arose to ask GPs for their views on the incidence and causes of infertility in their practice, and for information on their management practices and attitudes to the problem. This was conceived as a way of discovering the extent to which the experiences and attitudes related by couples in the clinic survey would be mirrored in what GPs themselves said about the same issues.

SOCIAL WORK AND CHILDLESSNESS

The childless have, so far, figured little more in social work literature, than in the other social sciences. As has been pointed out, the principal exception to this has been the attention paid to couples without children as a source of adoptive and foster homes, available to offer substitute family care to those children requiring such a service.

Traditionally, there has been a clear distinction between adoption and fostering (Heywood 1978). Adoption was seen as the permanent replacement of parents by substitutes, where the natural parents were unable or unwilling to care for the child in the long term. Adoption was, in most cases, a service provided by the childless married couple for illegitimate children. Foster care was, however, seen as the preserve of the 'experienced' couple, who had demonstrated their suitability in the raising of their own children. Recent developments in the provision of substitute family care have served to blur the distinctions between these roles (Smith 1984).

In recent years, there has been a drastic fall in the number of babies available for adoption by the infertile. Effective contraception is widely available. Unmarried mothers are less subject to social disapproval. Remarriage of those divorced or widowed has become common, providing continuing care for dependent children. Financial support has improved for single parents and their children. The provision of monetary help to prevent unnecessary receptions into care via Section 1 of the Children and Young Persons Act 1963 (replaced by Children Act 1989) might also have played a significant role in recent years. Adult adopted children, since the Children Act 1975, have had access to their birth records ending permanent separation from birth parents. Abortion of unwanted pregnancies has become readily available; in 1969, 53,000 abortions were performed under the Abortion Act 1967; in 1989, 184,000. The increase of abortions performed on unmarried women in particular has been very marked; the group which has in the past provided most of those babies adopted by the childless. In 1971, 46 per cent of abortions were performed on never-married women; by 1987 the proportion had risen to 60 per cent (OPCS 1988).

The combined effect of these changes has been to reduce drastically the number of babies becoming available for adoption by unrelated families. In 1974, 22,502 adoption orders were made; this fell to 10,240 in 1982 and 7,044 in 1989, including just 1,115 children aged under 1 (OPCS 1991).

In the wake of this sharp reduction in the 'supply' of children have come increasing hurdles erected by adoption agencies to reduce the imbalance between 'supply' and 'demand': residence and religious qualifications; age limits; requirements to have undergone *and completed* exhaustive testing; restricting the number of children to be placed to two or even one (Smith 1984, BAAF 1984).

Foster care has also undergone substantial changes. In recent years the number of children in the care of the local authorities has fluctuated. Rising to a high point of 95,300 for England in 1980, the numbers have fallen back to 74,900 in 1988. However, the numbers of children boarded out in foster care have risen, in both absolute and relative terms; from 28,400 or 32 per cent in 1973, to 34,600 or 46.2 per cent in 1988 (Department of Health 1989). The costs of residential care have also increased very sharply; the most recent available official estimate (CIPFA 1990) puts the average cost of residential care for children in a community home in England and Wales at £337.21 per child/week. At the same time, the literature casting severe doubt on the adequacy of non-family based, institutional care has grown. This literature saw the coming together of two distinct, but complementary, strands: the 'anti-institutional' literature (e.g. Goffman 1961, Townsend 1964, Wing and Brown 1970); and the psychoanalytically influenced literature concerning the essential attributes of 'good enough parenting' (e.g. Bowlby 1965, Newson and Newson 1965, Winnicott 1965). The combined effect of these factors was to see public and professional policy move towards the expansion of traditional and non-traditional approaches to fostering. Financial exigencies during the recession of the 1970s gave the impetus to this development, and it became commonplace for schemes to be promoted for placing children in foster care who would previously have been considered 'unfosterable' (see Cooper 1978, Triseliotis 1980).

The research study, *Children Who Wait* (Rowe and Lambert 1973), was particularly influential in encouraging social workers and their employing agencies to seek family placements wherever possible in place of residential care. This was envisaged as the way to offer children in care long-term security.

Alongside the extension of concepts of fosterability went a similar process with regard to adoption. Children previously felt to be unplaceable, or at best 'hard to place' (Sawbridge 1980), were placed in adoptive homes. The successful action research projects of the Parents for Children Project, and the Kent and Lambeth Family Placement Projects (Cooper 1978, Triseliotis 1980) were especially influential in demonstrating the possible achievements of this approach.

The combined effects for childless people have therefore been declining opportunities to adopt 'ordinary' babies and, simultaneously, a sense of pressure to consider the adoption of children with very different qualities and needs to those envisaged in a child of their own, at least before the discovery of their infertility. This could well add a further, difficult dimension to the relationships of social workers and childless people.

> To face childlessness is hard enough in itself; to then find oneself being made to feel guilty for not leaping with enthusiasm at the prospect of a mixed race or handicapped 'older child' is an unnecessary burden.
>
> (Sanderson 1985)

With the exception of Carole R. Smith's book (1984: 25–7) and Rowe's handbook for adoption workers, *Parents, Children and Adoption* (1966: 160–8), the emphasis in the adoption literature is to consider the childless almost exclusively from the point of view of their availability or suitability as prospective adoptive or foster parents. Indeed, a survey of the indices of a shelf of social workbooks on adoption, revealed only a very few with an entry for either infertility or childlessness. Jane Rowe in her influential guide for adoptive parents, *Yours by Choice*, interestingly entitles the section on these issues 'Do you really want to be a parent?'.

> All serious discussions about the success and failure of adoption place-
> ments are apt to come back again and again to the parents' feelings about
> their inability to have their own children. Until they can be comfortable
> about this, parents cannot be comfortable about an adopted child, for the
> child is a constant reminder of something they are trying to forget.
>
> (Rowe 1969: 35)

Amongst adoption officers and adoption agencies, there is a clear sense of priority in relation to their task. The following letter gives an illustration of this attitude, which is perhaps more often felt than expressed as baldly as in this case:

> Dear Editor,
>   'Fewer children were available for adoption in 1980 . . . the Church of
> England Children's Society has said . . . This has led to a drop in the
> number of children available to place with childless couples' (*News*,
> March 3).
>   If this is what the Church of England Children's Society actually said,
> I feel saddened that a society whose main concern is the child in need,
> perpetuates the implication that adoption is answering the needs of the
> childless couple.
>
> (Reid 1981)

There is no disputing the legal correctness of this position, but it perhaps typifies an attitude that the two concerns cannot be seen as complementary. Such negative expressions suggest that the social stigma of infertility is still extant, even amongst social workers.

Texts on social work in medical care either fail to identify the infertile as a group of patients requiring the services of the social worker (e.g. Davidson and Clarke 1989) or portray infertility as an example of a medical condition having a major psychosomatic component, only thus meriting the attention of the social worker (Butrym and Horder 1983: 64–5).

Two recent books have at last directed the attention of social workers to the predicament of childless people (Shapiro 1988, Valentine 1988). The issues addressed are those upon which this study was designed to cast light: the possible effects of infertility on the individual (e.g. grief, loss, anger, bereavement, confusion) and their relationships (marital, sexual). These and earlier contributions advocate the intervention of social workers; the modes of intervention discussed are principally counselling/casework and groupwork. Shapiro also discusses the contribution of training in assertiveness and problem-solving skills.

There is regular mention in this literature of the potential value of counselling, often referred to as brief or supportive psychotherapy, as an adjunct to the treatment of infertility (e.g. Karahasanoglu *et al.* 1972, Menning 1980, Philipp and Carruthers 1981, Shapiro 1988). Much of the literature on the possible psychogenic causes of infertility concludes with advocating such a service (Edelmann and Connolly 1986, Daniluk *et al.* 1987). Organisations for the childless, the National Association for the Childless and Child in the UK as well as Resolve in the United States, see the provision of counselling as amongst their primary concerns. The practitioners referred to in this context are not usually social workers, although social workers are prominent in the membership and management of all the 'self-help' groups mentioned. Two studies (Taylor 1982, Pepperell and McBain 1985) maintain the effectiveness of group counselling in promoting pregnancy amongst attenders of infertility clinics; however, their samples are so small and their manner of recruitment so selective that, despite their own conviction, their conclusions must be regarded as tentative. Edelmann and Connolly (1986) correctly observe the lack of any systematic appraisal of the efficacy of attempts to help the childless in this way, concluding:

> Most of the literature on infertility counselling, which is limited both in size and scope, is based upon assertions from counsellors rather than any systematic evaluation of the problems experienced by couples and methods employed to resolve them.

Since the completion of this study the case for counselling has gained acceptance through the recommendations of the Warnock Report (1984) and the pressure exerted by patient and interest groups, particularly the National Association for the Childless. The British Infertility Counselling Association was formed in 1988 to press for this service to be more widely available. The Human Fertilisation and Embryology Act 1990 accepted this consensus by requiring that infertility clinics make counselling available for couples accepted for treatment (*N.B.* only couples are mentioned).

Childless women have always been a prominent group amongst both residential and field social workers, perhaps the largest single group for much of social work's history. However, other than in the ways outlined above, childlessness has only recently been identified as an issue with which they should be concerned.

NOTE ON FIGURES AND STATISTICS

In the presentation of findings from the Clinic study the crude number of respondents will be given and also, in brackets, the percentage (rounded to the nearest whole number) in order to make immediately apparent the size relationship of the various subgroups to be discussed and the incidence of the characteristic of interest. The Clinic study group size is thirty in every case, unless an alternative '*N*' is given. In the case of the study of general practitioners (FPS) the sample size to which the percentage figures refer is 133, unless otherwise stated. The figures from the General Practice Study (GPS) will, where relevant, indicate the size of sample to which the percentage refers.

The *average* quoted will be the *mean*, unless otherwise stated. Where a *comparative population figure* is quoted, this is obtained from the General Household Survey 1981 (GHS), the Census 1981 (C), Social Trends (ST), Marriage and Divorce Statistics 1981 (MDS) or Birth Statistics 1981 (BS), all referenced under the Office of Population Censuses and Surveys (OPCS), their publisher. These figures refer to England and Wales, unless an alternative population is quoted.

Where a statement of statistical significance is made, this will be given as, e.g. $P = 0.045$, which indicates that the probability of such a finding would not be expected to occur by chance more often than 45 times in a thousand, or 4.5 per cent. Unless specifically mentioned, significance will not be suggested in cases where the test used does not achieve a level of confidence exceeding 95 per cent, that is an observed significance at 5 per cent, the level most commonly used in studies of this sort. The tests used are chi-square distribution (χ^2), Spearman's correlation coefficient (τ_s) or the two-sample *T*-test (*T*).

2 Understanding childlessness

It is difficult to identify with certainty those who are childless. The study of the different facets of childlessness is thus complicated and far from conclusive. This chapter will consider briefly what is known about its incidence (how common is it?), its causes, and its impact on those affected.

HOW COMMON IS CHILDLESSNESS?

There are a number of sources of information available as to the frequency with which childlessness might be found in a community. The fact that no one source is available to give definitive information was one of the motivating factors in this research.

Surveys that have sought the views of those anticipating marriage suggest that the vast majority expect parenthood (Woolf 1971, Dunnell 1979). The numbers of those who expect to have no children at all is consistently very low (Veevers 1979, 4.8 per cent; United Nations 1976, 0.5 per cent; Peel and Carr 1975, 4 per cent; Busfield and Paddon 1977, 5 per cent). Some of those intending to have no children will have medical reasons for the 'choice' – that is, probably, 'no choice'. As Cartwright (1976) notes, the evidence, such as it is, suggests that not only do intentions with regard to children vary over time in a marriage, but the decision to have another child is very much affected by a wide range of personal and 'public' experiences and attitudes, which is not fixed, but shifts and changes. In particular, an intention to have x children at the time of marriage, is a poor guide to completed family size.

A variety of studies have been conducted in Europe and North America which have produced rates of impaired fertility amongst married women between 9 and 22 per cent (e.g. Woolf 1971, Mazor and Simons 1984), and 8.5 per cent of all married couples (Hirsch and Mosher 1987).

The only epidemiological study of fertility in the community, available at the time of this research, was conducted in Denmark by Rachootin and

Olsen (1981). From a survey of 709 women aged 25–45, they found that 9 per cent had experienced 'reduced fecundity', i.e. failure to conceive during two years trying for a pregnancy. In a recent survey based on the operation of an infertility service in the West Country (Hull *et al.* 1985), an estimate is made of 1 in 6 couples, or 17 per cent needing infertility help at some time during the marriage.

Unfortunately the wealth of demographic evidence available in the UK does not provide clear answers: it tends to focus on households and can make no clear statement on the voluntary/involuntary 'distinction' mentioned already. Added to this is the finding (depressing to demographers) that as many as 20 per cent of those responding to the UK Census as 'childless', do in fact have children they did not record on their forms. Having no children at any point in time is no guide as to intentions, within child-bearing years at least.

Overall, there is consistent information suggesting that some 10 per cent of couples may remain childless, and that half of these will be experiencing a problem of impaired fertility. However, the difficulties of making precise and definitive measurements should not be underestimated.

IS CHILDLESSNESS INCREASING?

It is frequently suggested that childlessness is a growing phenomenon. Veevers (1972, 1980) and Baum (1980) point out that childlessness appeared to reach a peak in the depression years of the 1920s and 1930s, before falling substantially to very low rates in the post-war years. Farid (1974) and Veevers (1980) point to an increase in the rates more recently. Only at the age of menopause can completed fertility be measured, so it will be some time before the nature of this trend can be certainly stated. There are a number of factors which have been identified as possibly causing such a rise.

The age at which women are seeking to have their first child is one of the most commonly cited reasons. Age is well established as being negatively correlated with fertility. After a period in which women were marrying younger, it appears that this trend is changing. Women are marrying later, and delaying a first birth longer (OPCS 1990). The combined effect of such changes might well be to raise the overall rate of childlessness in the population.

James (1986) suggests that there is a biological decline in 'fecundability', evidenced by the 40 per cent decrease in non-identical twin births during the years 1960–80. Interpretation of these data is made very difficult by the increase in multiple births associated with the use of the modern reproductive technologies, which, to some extent deliberately, attempt to improve their success rates by causing super-ovulation and multiple embryo replacements (ILA 1990). All of James' papers readily acknowledge that the statistical sources of this information are not very reliable. James (1986) also claims that there was a measurable decline in sperm quality during the 1960s and 1970s in some parts of the world, including Europe. The extent to which these factors might affect the completed fertility rates of population in our society is, as yet, unknown.

Contraceptive practice plays a controversial role in fertility. Vessey *et al.* (1986) suggest that there is some negative impact of the contraceptive pill on fertility, particularly for childless women in their thirties. Two controversial contraceptive drugs have particularly been implicated in increased risk of infertility in the taker or her daughters; Depo Provera and DES (diethylstilbestrol) (Spallone 1989). The contraceptive practice to be most frequently blamed for causing infertility is the intrauterine device (IUD) (Anderson 1985).

There are various ways in which iatrogenic infertility might arise, that is, as an unwanted side effect of other medical interventions. Keye (1982) details the various surgical procedures which might inadvertently lead to impaired fertility. It is not clear that this is increasing, but Keye suggests that this is likely as the general rate of surgical intervention increases. It could also be argued that awareness of the dangers has made surgeons much more careful when conducting, for instance, appendicectomies on nulliparous women. Specialists in reproductive medicine do not seem to be optimistic that general surgery is necessarily less damaging, citing the continuing evidence of women having 'ovarian cysts' removed which prove to be corpus luteum.

In this category might also be placed the chemical hazards; hypotensive drugs and those used for the treatment of anxiety and depression have all been implicated in reduced fertility; all these classes of drugs have been increasingly prescribed in recent years. In addition, the illicit drugs of abuse, together with coffee, alcohol and tobacco, have all been linked to impaired fertility, acting by direct pharmacological action and through the reduction of sex drive (Denber 1978, Stanway 1980). Other environmental toxins, including radiation, have come under suspicion as causing more women to experience difficulty in conceiving or bearing live children (Spallone 1989).

Environmental pollutants may also be a factor, although the evidence is as yet limited. Smoking tobacco is known to have a deleterious effect on fertility (Howe *et al.* 1985) although smoking is currently a declining habit in all social groups (CSO 1989). Marijuana and numerous medically prescribed drugs, as mentioned above, have also been implicated in reduced fertility. Exposure to lead, iron, zinc or copper and to radiation or toxic fumes are all said to affect fertility in men (Stanway 1980: 160). The debate about the effects of food additives has also encompassed fertility (Hanssen 1984).

Abortion may also be of significance. The rate of induced abortion continues to rise: one-third of pregnancies established by women under the age of 20 in 1987 were ended by legally induced abortion (CSO 1989). The importance of abortion for subsequent fertility is controversial. Evidence suggests that where the procedure is carried out under optimal conditions using the latest techniques, the chance of secondary infections, which are of particular concern for future fertility, is greatly reduced (Cooke 1976). Stanway suggests (1980: 90) that the infertility risks of a properly carried out abortion are less than half those of a completed pregnancy.

Changing attitudes may also be of importance here. This issue will be discussed in detail in Chapter 3, 'Pronatalism'. As in other areas of social behaviour, it is argued that voluntary childlessness might be increasing as the shackles of social convention are loosened (Porter 1980). The analogy is made with the continuing steep rise in births outside marriage, now 25.6 per cent (OPCS 1990). Not only might more couples feel able to choose to have no children (Veevers 1980, Baum 1980) but other couples might feel less constrained to seek medical help for a failure to conceive (Pfeffer and Woollett 1983), or indeed less inclined to use scarce medical resources for this purpose (Parkes 1985). It must be acknowledged that assertion of 'the woman's right to choose' in this context might on the other hand substantially increase those who feel able to demand resources for the investigation of infertility (Spallone 1989).

A higher proportion of women are working outside the home, and more of them full time, than before. Childless women record higher rates of economic activity than mothers, although much of this difference must be accounted for by their greater availability. In their discussion of voluntary childlessness both Baum (1980) and Porter (1980) note the importance of the commitment to career in influencing child-bearing decisions. Again, this might also be a factor that interacts with age and delayed family formation to increase involuntary childlessness.

Increased educational achievement is well recognised as a consistent correlate of childlessness. More women are achieving higher levels than before, which is clearly related on past experience to lower fertility. Of those women born between 1935 and 1939, 16 per cent with 'O'levels and above remained childless, but only 8 per cent of the others (OPCS 1989). This factor is likely to interact in the same way with age and delayed family building, and also to have an impact on rates of involuntary childlessness.

Increased levels of stress may play a part. Whether or not it is valid to claim higher rates of stress for our current society is also a highly contentious issue. It is conventional to claim increased rates of stress for modern western industrial society, but one might question whether or not this is again an example of

> the hypochondria of moralists who diagnose a diseased present because they worship a past they do not understand.

(McGregor 1957)

as well as a form of ethnocentrism that fails to recognise, or evaluate correctly, the stresses encountered by other cultures. However, it is common for writers on infertility to cite stress as a cause of increasing rates of infertility (e.g. Stangel 1979, Stanway 1984).

Sexually transmitted diseases may be playing an increasingly important role. Venereal disease, gonorrhoea, and chlamydia trachomatis infections are believed to be particularly implicated in infertility; all treatable but underdiagnosed problems according to Diczfalusy (1986).

Stanway, reviewing some of the evidence presented here, suggests that the proportion of infertile people in the UK and in the west as a whole will almost certainly rise to over 20 per cent in the next decade or two (Stanway 1980).

Together with the hypothesised increase in voluntary childlessness (Veevers 1980), this would amount to a massive decrease in overall population fertility. This apocalyptic view appears to be slightly less appropriate now, than it did at the beginning of the 1980s. From the low point of 1977, when the general fertility rate was 58.2, it rose to 63.0 in 1988 (total births per 1,000 women aged 15–44, OPCS 1990). Total period fertility rate, at 1.82, is still below the level of replacement, 2.1.

Demographic conditions are undoubtedly more propitious for the resourcing of infertility investigation than they have been. The increasing efficacy of medical treatment, and the massive strides that have been made in scientific understanding of the reproductive processes, might, however, serve to off-set these factors which are tending to raise rates of infertility.

Our knowledge is still too scant to answer this question with certainty: however, childlessness is certainly more common than was once thought.

WHAT CAUSES INFERTILITY?

The causes of infertility are many, and the state of medical knowledge is constantly improving. The last decade has been a period of perhaps unprecedented growth in the understanding of the problems associated with reproduction and fertility. Consequently, the range of available treatments has also grown substantially. As mentioned previously, it might be the case that the dramatic decline in the birth rate precipitated some of these developments, if not directly, at least by creating the climate in which there is greater sympathy towards the claims of this group of people for medical attention than has hitherto been the case.

It would not be appropriate here to give great detail of the nature of the many medical problems associated with infertility. A glossary of the more significant conditions, with brief explanations, is available as Appendix IV. The matters of particular interest here are those of unexplained infertility and psychogenic, or functional, infertility. Both of these arouse considerable controversy.

Some comment might be made on the relative frequency of the different causes of infertility, in order to put the discussion of psychological factors in context.

Medical factors

As there have been no epidemiological studies of the relative frequency of occurrence of the disorders associated with infertility, the available evidence derives from the analysis of data obtained by infertility treatment services in their clinical practice. The rates obtained will therefore say as much about the interests and the catchment area of the clinic as the real incidence of the problems (Cooke 1976).

From a general review of the available evidence (Thomas and Forrest 1980, Hull *et al.* 1985, Wren 1985) it seems that the most frequent causes of infertility are sperm defects, ovulatory disorders and tubal problems. However, it is important to keep in mind that with improved measurement techniques come changes in the evaluation of fertility status. It is frequently pointed out that sperm viability is particularly poorly understood. Studies of vasectomy samples of males of known fertility show that some men achieve pregnancies in their partners with sperm samples that would be regarded as subfertile if evaluated by an infertility service (Stanway 1980). Similarly, the assessment of adequate ovulation has changed substantially in recent years. The endocrinology of ovulation can detect more subtle difficulties which, in the past, would have led to a diagnosis of unexplained infertility (Lenton *et al.* 1977).

All specialists in reproductive medicine (recently approved as a subspecialism by the Royal College of Obstetricians and Gynaecologists) would agree that there is a great deal yet to be learned about the causes and treatment of infertility. Research has been particularly slow in the area of male infertility. Whilst it is still the case, as is common knowledge, that 'more can be done' for the woman than the man, this situation may change.

Should population fertility continue at a level below replacement in western societies, then this factor might replace the pressure to limit population growth in determining the attitudes of medical research to human infertility. The recommendations of the Warnock Report (1984) and the Human Fertilisation and Embryology Act 1990 might be said to be evidence of such a change. The search for improved contraceptives has already been a fruitful source of knowledge for this field, and is likely to continue to be so. These changed social conditions might encourage application of this knowledge directly to the needs of the infertile.

Psychological factors

The concern here is with the role of psychological factors in the causation of infertility, rather than with the role these factors play in the way people cope with their impaired fertility. This is an area of considerable controversy which is fuelled by the enormous methodological problems posed in trying to investigate this factor. As has been mentioned elsewhere, without sound, prospective, epidemiological studies of couples, some of whom will become infertile, it is very difficult to disentangle cause and effect. There is no doubt that being infertile is experienced by many as a most distressing situation, and there is substantial anecdotal and psychological evidence, discussed below, which confirms this. However, the importance of these factors in *causing* infertility is much less clear. The literature suggesting an etiological role for personality or emotional factors has to rely on data gleaned from those who have already identified themselves as having a fertility problem, and have been referred for specialist investigation. Consequently, such studies are vulnerable to charges of claiming as causative those experiences which are, in reality, reactive to the stressful situation of infertility: the chicken or egg problem. In reporting the experiences of an unselected group of infertility patients, this book will help untangle this problem.

Several terms have been used to cover this area of concern: psychosomatic, psychogenic or functional infertility. All refer to the same proposition, that there is a group of patients whose infertility is primarily caused by psychological factors in the broadest sense – that is, there is either no physiological cause at all, or only physiological factors which have been triggered by a psychological condition. I shall use the term functional here for these situations.

There are several areas in which it is suggested that there is evidence for functional infertility.

Firstly, there are those writers who claim that it is possible to identify a group of infertile people (usually women) who have *personality problems*. It is of interest that the greater part of this literature is written by men and refers to women. Writers have been much less ready to ascribe defective personalities to infertile men. This has caused feminist writers to be particularly critical of this approach (e.g. Pfeffer and Woollett 1983, Stanworth 1987). Most of the 'evidence' derives from small numbers of case histories described by psychoanalytically trained psychiatrists or psychologists working on referral from gynaecologists, (e.g. Norris 1965, Ladeira 1977). Raphael-Leff (1990) comments that

> The identity of some women is so embedded in having a baby that they cannot envisage themselves except as mothers. [A woman may become pregnant on] discovering her own identity and finding that she can face life even if she does not have a child.

This argument is that some infertile women, whilst apparently obsessively seeking help, unconsciously fear sexual intercourse and reject the very ideas of pregnancy, childbirth, and motherhood.

The fewer papers on men, focusing on impotence, reflect a similar approach (e.g. Abse 1966, Noy *et al.* 1966, Palti 1969). This is interpreted as reflecting the unresolved oedipal drive of repressed sexual attraction to the mother. The necessity to repress this incestuous desire leads to fears of castration and to impotence, its behavioural manifestation. Secondary to this, is posited the unconscious desire to punish the wife for daring to assume the place of the mother.

Denber, in his review of these approaches, puts the central criticism pungently:

> I cannot find any evidence that controlled studies have been brought forward to validate the hypothesis. It is one thing to firmly 'believe' something and another to have 'firm proof' of the facts.
>
> (Denber 1978)

Without evidence from carefully constructed studies, which psychodynamic investigators invariably decline to undertake (Eysenck 1986), these ideas should be treated with scepticism. Yet their influence is plain, although unacknowledged:

> With some other women, personality disorders are more deep-seated. (They) have obsessional or downright aggressive personalities, and . . . make themselves infertile by their temperaments . . . Aggressive women are the most difficult to deal with because they rapidly antagonise every doctor with whom they come into contact. Recently, a woman 'phoned me to ask for an appointment. While I was trying to get details of her problem she took me by surprise by accusing me of inconsistency in that I was saying the opposite of what I had written in some previous article. I tried to give her an explanation but she became quite hysterical and,

sobbing, screamed 'Oh God! You are no use to anyone!' and slammed down the receiver. I doubt if any doctor could help this sad woman. She is the victim of her own personality.

(Newill 1981)

This article is quoted at some length, as it appears to demonstrate the effect this approach can have on the attitudes of at least one male doctor. In this article, Dr Newill is supposedly reviewing the evidence for functional infertility, yet large sections of it are devoted to this sort of invective. This vein of argument has, arguably, done more to exacerbate relationships between doctors and their patients than it has elucidated the nature of their difficulties, appearing as it does to 'blame the victim'. Denber's criticism has been widely echoed in recent literature, and these articles seemed to be appearing with less frequency in the specialist press, although the upsurge of research prompted by the introduction of IVF treatment has included further material of this kind (Mazure and Greenfeld 1989).

Secondly, the role of *stress* in prejudicing fertility is more widely accepted. Interested readers can find the evidence reviewed in detail by Garcia *et al.* (1985), who conclude that only in the case of menstruation is there sometimes an unequivocal psychological cause. Conception cannot, of course, occur without menstruation. Many studies have been done which demonstrate that severe psychological distress can lead to periods ceasing or changing in character; depression and anorexia in young women are frequently cited. Stress might operate by increasing the level of prolactin in the blood to the point where menstruation is stopped (Harper *et al.* 1985), and is known to affect the endocrine system so crucial in the control of fertility. Severe externally generated stress is also believed to lead to impaired sperm production in men, although there is little recent evidence (Sand 1935, Stanway 1980). Assertions are made in the literature that emotional factors cause or contribute to anything between 4.3 per cent (Philipp and Carruthers 1981) and 25 per cent (Walker 1978) of infertility. Studies supporting a high incidence of these problems have signally failed to distinguish between emotional conditions identifiable before onset of infertility and that found where childlessness is already causing concern. Several investigators have claimed success for psychotherapy, individually or in groups, in enabling women with a fertility problem to become pregnant. Although the value of counselling is generally acknowledged in alleviating distress, the published studies (e.g. Taylor 1982) fail to prove that the distress helped in this way was a primary cause of the infertility. No conclusive evidence has been produced that a specific psychological factor can alter fertility in the normal fertile couple (e.g. Mai *et al.* 1972, Freeman *et al.* 1983).

Thirdly, *sexual difficulties*, which prevent adequate intercourse, are known to be frequently psychological in origin. These are principally vaginismus or dyspareunia in women and impotence or premature ejaculation in men, which are accepted as having a substantial, and sometimes exclusive, psychological component (Stangel 1979). These appear to be comparatively uncommon causes of infertility as seen at infertility clinics. No doubt this reflects the fact that the couple concerned are unlikely not to have a good idea of the cause of their difficulty, and, if wishing it to be treated, are likely to seek treatment for that condition. Most of those so affected may be seen elsewhere, e.g. Relate (Marriage Guidance Councils). Simple sexual ignorance may be the cause, or a side effect of various drugs (see Bancroft 1983).

Fourthly, the '*waiting list effect*' has been used in support of these views. A not inconsiderable number of patients do conceive whilst on the waiting list for referral to the infertility service, or during investigation but prior to any active treatment. That some women should become pregnant whilst awaiting investigation appears less surprising if one looks at the time taken to achieve pregnancy. Cartwright, in her study *How Many Children* (1976), found that 19 per cent of women (who had already given birth to a child) took one year or more to achieve the desired pregnancy, and 11 per cent took two years or more. The periods of unprotected intercourse to achieve pregnancy were strongly related to both the age of the mother and the length of marriage; half the mothers aged 35 and over and 58 per cent of those married 15 years or more took two years or more to conceive. Mazor and Simons (1984) suggest that, for all women, only four out of five will have conceived by the end of the first year of unrestricted intercourse: this is the 'normal' criterion used in determining that referral for investigation is appropriate (Jones 1991). In view of this evidence, the importance attached to the 'waiting list' factor seems inappropriate.

Fifthly, there is the matter of *unexplained infertility*: the existence of a substantial group whose infertility cannot be satisfactorily explained has been used to substantiate the view that functional infertility is a major factor. Hull *et al.* (1985) claim this represents 13 per cent of referrals. Lenton *et al.* (1977) found that 'the patients in our series [of diagnoses of unexplained infertility] do have some abnormality even though we have failed to demonstrate it'. They go on to point out the areas of investigation which had been inadequate, partly through the subsequent expansion of knowledge; these included estimation of pelvic pathology, immunologic factors and quality of ovulation. Further evidence that the category 'unexplained infertility' might be a euphemism for 'inadequate clinical investigation' was presented in a study by Winston (1990) of 100 couples referred for IVF treatment with this 'diagnosis', of whom he concluded only 6 per cent had been fully and adequately investigated. Burslem and Osborn (1986) conclude that

> in many cases a much more rigorous investigation of such couples will uncover reasons to explain the unexplained and may, thereby, provide at least some hope for rational and effective treatment in the future.

Sixthly, there is *post-adoption conception.* This is the commonly held belief, in lay and medical circles, that adopting couples, even after long periods of infertility investigation and treatment, and having been given little hope of conceiving their own child, still achieve conception once an adoptive child has been placed. I personally remember the discomfiture of a psychiatrist whose wife conceived in these circumstances. Kornitzer (1968) and Sandler (1965) have been influential in arguing that once the stress of failing to achieve the desired pregnancy is removed, the consequent relaxation permits conception. Parents, particularly adopters, may find the suggestion surprising that the arrival of a child in the family reduces stress in this way. The number of studies that have been done into this alleged phenomenon is, in itself, tribute to the tenacity of the idea. A review of this material suggests that we should conclude with Edelmann and Connolly (1986) that 'the speculation about the therapeutic value of adoption was unfounded'.

Over the years, the concept of functional infertility has come to occupy a significant position in any discussion of the causes of infertility. Some of the reasons for this have been discussed. Pfeffer and Woollett (1983: 47) dismiss the case thus: 'there is no good evidence to support the idea of the emotional or psychological causation of infertility.' Although they do not deploy the argument directly, it is implicitly accepted by these feminist writers, that this assertion might be regarded as further evidence of the sexism prevalent amongst male doctors that all too readily imputes emotional instability to their female patients (cf. Ehrenreich and English 1974, Chesler 1974).

Only by carefully conducted longitudinal studies will the relationship between infertility and psychopathology be satisfactorily investigated and disentangled. At the moment 'research has not identified psychological causes of infertility beyond amenorrhoea induced by stress, and so concern has shifted to emotional distress produced by infertility and its treatment' (Garcia *et al.* 1985).

The study group will offer important evidence as to the nature of the strains imposed by the experience of infertility and its treatment, which will contribute to the debate as to the importance of stress and anxiety in this condition. Following the patients over an extended period of time offers evidence as to the changes that occur in this area. The factors in the social

situation of the couple and in the nature of the infertility services available
to them, which, jointly or separately, contribute to their experience of stress
will become evident.

Emphasising the general level of anxiety experienced by these people
might serve to discourage those too ready to attribute psychological causes
to their problems in the absence of clear pathology. My purpose is not to
deny the importance of these issues. The danger is that they are used to
construct a residual etiological category, which indiscriminately conflates
cause and effect.

IMPACT OF CHILDLESSNESS

Such literature as is available, however, testifies to the extreme distress
caused to the individual and couple concerned, and the tension brought
about for their relationships. In most cases, it might be fair to say, this
distress is portrayed as very painful, but survivable.

Personal accounts

A rich source of such material lies in fiction and autobiographical accounts.
Silas Marner by George Eliot is one of the more significant treatments of
childlessness in literature. It runs as a theme throughout the novel: the
barren life of the solitary miser, Marner, made meaningful by the arrival in
his life of a little 'orphan' girl, Eppie; her golden hair he takes as divine
substitution for his stolen, earthly gold; Squire Pass is the natural father
who never openly acknowledged her; when it becomes clear in his second,
public marriage that he will otherwise remain childless, Squire and Mrs
Pass try to persuade Eppie to live with them; by this time Eppie will not
disown the 'father' who brought her up. The childlessness of the Passes is
portrayed as a wound which never heals.

> And Nancy's deepest wounds had all come from the perception that the
> absence of children from their hearth was dwelt on in her husband's
> mind as a privation to which he could not reconcile himself.
>
> (Eliot 1967: 215)

It may be no coincidence that *Silas Marner* is unusual amongst her novels
in the strong narrative line of plot it contains; and George Eliot (Mary Ann
Evans) never had children (Adam 1969).

Modern treatments of this situation include the novels of Nigel Balchin,
Mine Own Executioner (1945) and *A Way Through The Wood* (1951).
Three recent books stand out for their extended, frank discussion, in novel
form, of the pains of infertility and childlessness: *The Wife Wants a Child*

by Gwyneth Branfoot (1983); *The Daughters of Jerusalem* by Sara Maitland (1987); *Blizzard and the Holy Ghost* by Joseph Blizzard (1977).

> Oh Jesus, why did this have to happen? . . . All this time we've been waiting. We wanted kids so much, do you know that? Why couldn't we be like the rest of the world and just have them? All the rest of the bloody world can do it!.
>
> (Branfoot 1983: 103)

In the third of these books, Blizzard tells the story of infertility from the man's point of view. In the other two books the infertility was on the woman's side; in this case it is the man's sterility and his struggle to come to terms with it, and with its only remedy, donor insemination (DI), which provide the focus for the narrative. Although in the form of a novel, this is, in fact, autobiographical. The continued stigma attached to male infertility, which is arguably even greater than that experienced by the female, and the social stereotype of maleness that discourages discussion of infertility amongst those men affected, leads this author, a doctor, to write anonymously. The producers of a popular television programme on infertility in the *Bodymatters* series (BBC Television 8/9/86) claimed to have been unable to find an infertile man willing to be interviewed on the programme, as did Miall in her research into childlessness in Canada. Blizzard writes that 'childlessness would have been a greater price to pay than the difficulties described in this book' (Blizzard 1977: 17). Blizzard writes vividly of the personal doubt, the sense of failure, the insensitivity of doctors, the strain to the marriage and his personal resentment and bitterness. However, in the gradual acceptance of sterility, and then DI, the author says 'slowly the nightmare has become a dream' (Blizzard 1977: 178).

A particularly vivid account of the personal impact of infertility on a woman was given by Sylvia Plath, in her poem 'Childless Woman' (Plath 1981: 259). Although not apparently autobiographical – as Plath had two children, the first born four years after her marriage – the authenticity of this cry of desolation and agony suggests a personal commitment such as is found in so much of her poetry. Published biographies of the poet, her letters and the commentary of her husband, Ted Hughes, to the *Collected Poems* give no guidance as to whether the commitment in this poem is from personal or empathic experience or has a more symbolic content. Three months after writing this poem, the author killed herself.

Playwrights have produced several dramatically powerful evocations of the same subject. The most famous is undoubtedly Edward Albee's *Who's Afraid of Virginia Woolf?*, particularly in the film performance with Richard Burton as George and Elizabeth Taylor as Martha. The play recounts the battleground that their marriage has become; the utter hopelessness of reclaiming the experience of love between the partners. The central failure, childlessness, has sapped their relationship of all warmth and affection. Their desperation to produce a child, and the shared perception that, without a child, the marriage has no meaning – and nor have their own lives – leads them to produce a fantasy son. This son becomes the focus of all their frustration and antipathy, and, at the same time, the only spark of hope for themselves and their marriage. In a famous speech, Martha proclaims 'his' importance:

> The one thing I've tried to carry pure and unscathed through the sewer of this marriage; through the sick nights and the pathetic, stupid days, through the derision and the laughter . . . God, the laughter . . . through one failure after another, one failure compounding another failure, each attempt more sickening, more numbing than the one before; the one thing, the one person I have tried to protect, to raise above the mire of this vile, crushing marriage; the one light in all this hopeless . . . darkness . . . our SON.

> (Albee 1962: 132)

Yet the burden of their mutual despair becomes too much, and George, in a final fit of pique and self-destructive punishment, 'kills' this son off. This act is a sign, not of final reconciliation, but of final, irreconcilable despair.

Federico Garcia Lorca's rarely produced play 'Yerma' (Garcia Lorca 1987) uses the subject of childlessness as a metaphor for the powerlessness of women in Spanish society of the 1930s.

In David Rudkin's *Ashes* (1978) we follow the painful path of Colin and Anne in their attempts to conceive and the lengthy treatment they undergo. Two pregnancies miscarry and they are turned down for adoption, and the play reverberates with the agony, mental and physical, the humiliation, and the despair.

There has, in recent years, been a marked increase in the number of popular articles in the press and women's magazines concerning the pains of infertility. The burden of these articles has been the extent of the distress experienced by those who are involuntarily childless, and, in general terms, how little support they receive from 'clinical' doctors, thoughtless friends and family who do not know how to help with the hurt. Claire Rayner, one of the more thoughtful of the media 'agony aunts', has experienced the problem herself. She has written of the misery and worry and the damage caused in several areas: the self-image, sexuality, the relationship with the partner, and relationships with other people. An article in a newspaper in which a couple shared the depth of their own suffering, led to the foundation of the National Association for the Childless, which has played an important role in promoting publicity concerning these experiences and needs (Houghton and Houghton 1977, 1984).

The plight of the infertile has begun to appear on the television 'soap operas'; this is an indication that the issue is now being taken more seriously and is more socially acceptable (Eastenders 1988, The Archers 1989). Several books include real personal experiences of infertility, although none has attempted to collect such accounts systematically (Menning 1977, Stanway 1980, Pfeffer and Woollett 1983, Jones 1991). It is the lack of systematic evidence derived from research that part of this study was designed to fulfil.

Childless marriages

The personal accounts discussed above, and those to be found in Houghton and Houghton (1984) and Pfeffer and Woollett (1983), as well as in the pages of *NACK* and *Issue*, attest to the strains imposed on a marriage by involuntary childlessness. One measure of this strain might be the divorce rate. These studies have a persistent problem: they usually fail to, or cannot, distinguish between those who chose not to have children, or through disharmony did not have the opportunity, and those who could not have children.

In the last twenty years divorces have increased six times: 158,000 divorces were granted in 1984 (OPCS 1986c). Current projections suggest that as many as one in four of those who marry will have been divorced by the time they are 45. The relative proclivity of childless marriages and those with children to break down has for some time been a matter of debate. The proportion of divorcing couples without children has changed little in recent years, standing at 30.8 per cent in 1988 (OPCS 1989).

Hart notes that:

> The presence of children in the nuclear home may on the one hand help to create a closer identification of common interests between the two partners, and yet on the other be a source of friction and conflict.
>
> (Hart 1976: 78)

Brannen and Collard (1982) in their study *Marriages in Trouble* found substantial reluctance to consider divorce an acceptable resolution for marital discord where there were young children. The traditional attitude that marriages should continue 'for the sake of the children', unless there were considerable, damaging disharmony, appeared still to receive considerable support. Chester (1972), scrutinising this assumed association between childlessness and divorce, suggests that arguments for it include:

the negative effects of childlessness; the coalescing effects of children; latent homosexuality represented as infertility; selfishness; reduced commitment to marriage; repugnance towards child-bearing. These very personal attitudes suggest an affinity with the pronatalist pressures discussed elsewhere.

In the long-term follow-up of couples previously treated in an infertility clinic, for whom no conclusive diagnosis had been established, Lenton *et al.* (1977) found that only five out of 96 couples had divorced during the intervening years since discharge, a period of between four and nine years.

The significance of this often-reported correlation between childlessness and divorce has been disputed. Chester (1972) argued that the association often assumed is largely a product of faulty statistics, notably the failure to hold constant the length of marriage when conception was possible. Gibson (1980) and Chester both argue that other factors are of much greater significance in understanding the causes of marital breakdown, including the age of marriage, the length of courtship and socio-economic factors. Thornes and Collard (1979) note the impact of marital instability on sexual adjustment and opportunities for conception.

Pending further careful research, particularly longitudinal studies as advocated by Gibson, this association should be regarded as not proven.

Prior to the present study, there seems to have been no other attempt to monitor the effects of infertility on the marital relationship, as both evolved over an extended period of time. Comments on this matter have, therefore, been the result of practice observation and personal account or 'snapshot' studies, rather than systematic longitudinal study.

Edelmann and Connolly (1986) maintain that such evidence as is available suggests that infertility does have an impact on the marriage 'but that some couples adapt well to their childless state'. The results of a large postal survey of infertility patients support the view that infertility does increase the rate of marital problems for a couple, particularly where the fertility problem lies with the man (Connolly, *et al.* 1987). Other researchers, including Humphrey (1969) and Giele-Zwier (1971), report no significant increase in marital dissatisfaction amongst childless respondents. Veevers argues:

> In most instances available data suggest a positive correlation between childlessness and marital satisfaction.
>
> (Veevers 1979: 13)

However, Debrovner and Shubin-Stein (1976) reported marital difficulties both during, and subsequent to, the infertility investigation. This is confirmed in the rich anecdotal evidence offered by Menning (1977), Houghton and Houghton (1977, 1984) and Pfeffer and Woollett (1983).

Recent studies of marriage have identified high rates of difficulties in all marriages (e.g. Thornes and Collard 1979, Garde and Lunde 1980). Brannen and Collard (1982) studied *Marriages in Trouble*, but in no case did difficulties in having children figure as a precipitant, even amongst those without children. The striking feature of their report is that children hardly figure at all.

These sources of evidence do not appear to support the notion that childless marriages are peculiarly vulnerable to breakdown.

Studies of the impact of other forms of stressful experience on marriage, which might be said to have analogies with the experience of childlessness, seem also to support this positive view. Marriages which are, in interpersonal terms, stable seem able to cope under substantial levels of stress. Evidence for this position may be found in many studies, including Dominian (1968) on marital breakdown, Brown and Harris (1978) on depression, Korer and Fitzsimmons (1985) on Huntington's chorea, Hart (1976) on divorce, Voysey (1975) on families with a disabled child.

Evidence concerning the effects of childlessness on a marriage might also be derived from looking at the opposite situation; namely, the effects of children on a marriage. There is a clear tendency, in the older literature particularly, to mirror popular, pronatalist assumptions that marriages are invariably happier where there are children than where there are not. Dominian (1968: 96) claims that 'children bind their parents together in a common goal and purpose'. However, Jones (1967) reported almost half of her sample of 'new mothers' feeling that pregnancy had made their marriages *less* happy, rather than more happy, as pictured in romantic fiction. More recent literature tends to support this less positive view (Rollins and Cannon 1974, Campbell 1975, Brown and Harris 1978, Oakley 1979). Noting that 'a woman's involvement in her children can mean an emotional withdrawal from the marital relationship', Boulton (1983: 164) found that, for a quarter of her mothers, maternity had led to problems in the marriage.

Studies of the impact of children on marriage do not tend to support the view that they are invariably a positive force in the relationship, rather the reverse.

Psychological impact

As discussed in the context of evidence concerning the etiological factors of infertility, there is substantial confusion in the literature between cause and effect. The evidence for infertility being *caused* by psychological or emotional factors is not substantial, although the evidence for infertility having a profound but non-specific psychological and emotional *effect* is.

Garcia *et al.* (1985) claim that research has failed to identify psychological causes of infertility beyond amenorrhoea induced by stress, so concern has shifted to the emotional distress produced by infertility and its treatment.

Personal functioning

There have been few well-designed studies to investigate the impact of infertility on psychological functioning, although there is a wide measure of agreement that the impact is substantial. The interested reader may find these discussed in detail by Edelmann and Connolly (1986) and Monach (1987). As the former observe:

> The impact of infertility upon psychological functions is a complex matter influenced by many variables including the duration of infertility, the investigative procedures carried out, whether the cause of infertility is with the man or the woman, and the diagnosis and prognosis from the investigations.
>
> (Edelmann and Connolly 1986)

To this list might be added variables such as the previous relationship and personality, social and economic factors, and the clinical regime to which they are subjected. The complexity of this task should not be underestimated.

From a survey of infertility clinic patients, Connolly *et al.* (1987) found:

> Overall there is a general tendency for an extended period of investigation to lead to an increase in distress scores for women . . . Feelings of hopelessness and despair, and consequent depression, are likely to increase as the failure cycle is repeated month by month.

The consensus of commentators appears to remain that whilst personal accounts and anecdotal evidence point to the great psychological pressures faced by those unable to conceive a child, there is not, as yet, sound research evidence as to the exact nature of the supposed psychological problems. Mai (1972) characterised the situation as 'an absence of information . . . more than counterbalanced by a surfeit of hypotheses'. This does not ignore the strong evidence already mentioned for the extent of distress suffered by the childless, which is discussed further below.

Sexual functioning

There is little disagreement in the literature that the sexual relationship of the infertile couple is likely to be affected.

Most couples undergoing investigations and treatment and the stages of emotional reaction along to the final diagnosis of infertility suffer a body blow to their sexual relationship.

(Stanway 1980: 168)

The debate involves the extent to which sexual difficulties might be considered to precede the infertility, and actually cause it. Philipp and Carruthers (1981) suggest that between 5 and 10 per cent of infertile couples will include an individual unable to consummate intercourse, of whom some will have psychogenic causes and some physical, and there may be no clear dividing line between the two. There are a number of situations in this category of potential causes of infertility.

Impotence amongst men is cited as a frequent matter of concern. By this is meant either the inability to achieve and sustain an erection sufficient to achieve full penetration of the vagina, or premature ejaculation. In either case conception is unlikely to occur. Impotence has no necessary connection with fertility, in the sense that a man might well have semen within normal limits of fertility and yet be impotent. Indeed, this will normally be the case. However, it is often suggested that in the popular mind there is believed to be a close connection between the two. This was borne out in this study. Miall (1986: 274) notes that:

male infertility [was considered] more discrediting to masculinity than female infertility to femininity, and [they] associated male infertility with impotence or a lack of virility.

Both physical and psychological causes are known for this condition. Physical factors include: diabetes; drugs used for hypertension and anxiety; oestrogens used in cancer and severe acne treatment; tumours; and degenerative illnesses, such as multiple sclerosis, affecting the central nervous system. There may be hormonal defects, in a reduced level of testosterone, the male sex-related hormone.

On the other hand, the impotence might arise without apparent physical cause as a result of stress and anxiety (see Fischer and Gochros 1977 and Kaplan 1978). It is usually reported in the context of established marriages, in which their fertility status is not seen as being of central concern, the marriages having already produced children. In such cases the impotence is most often reported as having its origin in environmental stresses of occupation, financial resources and relationships, although there is also extensive discussion in the psychiatric literature of those origins in personal and psycho-sexual development (e.g. Storr 1964).

Difficulty with intercourse may be an important contributor to infertility problems. The principal conditions here are dyspareunia (pain during intercourse) and vaginismus (vaginal spasm prior to/during intercourse). Causes for these two conditions include those of physical origin (infection, inflammation) and others of psychological origin (fear of intercourse, reaction to rape). It is important to recognise the interaction of both sorts of explanation. Frigidity would in the past have figured in a discussion of this sort, but the term has been debased in usage, attracting a sexist, pejorative connotation and is better avoided in favour of specific terms denoting the precise form of dysfunction; for example, the avoidance of intercourse due to pain, or distaste, or orgasmic dysfunction, etc.

Orgasmic dysfunction may contribute to infertility in the woman, although this is a matter of some debate. (In the man, of course, orgasm is essential for natural conception, although pregnancy may still be achieved through artificial insemination by husband, AIH.) Although obviously hard to measure, as many as one in seven women never experience orgasm during sexual intercourse (Gebhard and Johnson 1979). Some authors assert that orgasm in the woman performs a reproductive function, in that it increases the receptivity of the genital tract to the sperm and aids the progress of the sperm by the creation of negative pressure in the uterus (Stanway 1980). However, orgasm is plainly not essential for conception, given the large number of women who conceive without ever, apparently, experiencing orgasm. It might be expected to become more crucial in circumstances of reduced fertility. The literature seems to discount the possibility of there frequently being found a physiological basis for the failure of orgasm, concentrating rather on the importance of psycho-social factors related to the development of attitudes to sex, early experience of sex, attitudes to the sexual partner, and the nature of the current sexual relationship(s) (Brecher and Brecher 1966).

Sexual ignorance is frequently mentioned in texts concerning medical practice in infertility, and instruction in sexual technique forms a significant part of those books on the subject aimed at a lay audience. In general discussion, gynaecologists frequently relate the appearance in their clinics of couples who have failed to consummate the relationship, whilst believing themselves to be having a normal sex life: some 'infertile' women are actually virgins. In these so-called 'permissive' days, the extent of sexual ignorance is surprising.

Sexual attitudes/dissatisfaction may be of particular concern in understanding the genesis of an infertility problem. Studies reviewed by Bancroft (1983) emphasise the widespread nature of dissatisfaction with the sexual relationship between husband and wife unaffected by infertility. Estimates are given ranging from 12 to 26 per cent of men and 9 per cent to 43 per cent of women.

Whether or not we accept the central importance of mature sexuality to personality development asserted by Freudians, I would support Menning's argument that failure to create a sound sense of self-esteem which incorporates a realistic and secure self-image, particularly in relation to sexuality, will make one especially vulnerable if there is an infertility problem (Menning 1977: ch. 13). This is the case in our society *a fortiori* because of the continuing pronatalist pressure, discussed in the next chapter, which identifies sexuality so closely with the ability to reproduce. It will be seen that one of the couples involved in this study clearly had unusual and negative attitudes to sexuality, although the relevance of this to their infertility problem was not clearly etiological. The psychoanalytic literature typified by Deutsch (1945) stresses the importance of defective development in this area for the onset of infertility. As described above, the evidence for this position, in properly controlled studies of representative infertile women, has so far not emerged as it relies entirely on small numbers of case studies. There is little doubt that sexual adjustment does suffer with the identification and treatment of infertility, and a number of studies have confirmed this.

Those sources of personal accounts of infertility which have already been extensively cited, all contain substantial testimony to the sexual difficulties which were experienced in these circumstances (Menning 1977, Houghton and Houghton 1977, 1984, Pfeffer and Woollett 1983). The focus in these accounts is particularly on the extent to which this private activity is subjected to the scrutiny of a third party, the doctor, in ways which are never endured by most couples. The sense of privacy which surrounds sex has not very substantially been eroded by the increased public attention given to the matter with the 'permissive society'. Menning describes this graphically as the *ménage à trois*, or three in the bed:

> A man, a woman and a thermometer make strange bedfellows. The act of charting each day of the menstrual cycle and each sexual encounter focusses attention morbidly on infertility and the attempts to overcome it. Converting sexual relations to little X's on a chart also makes public something that most couples consider very private and do not ordinarily keep a score on. 'We felt like we always had someone between the sheets with us. First and foremost there was the thermometer. Then the doctor. We felt at various times as if both sets of our parents were in the bed with us. And finally, during adoption, the social worker seemed to join us in the bed. During this whole time we have never had that bed to ourselves.'
>
> (Menning 1977: 126)

The importance attached to the correct timing of intercourse at the most fertile period of the woman's menstrual cycle is a central feature of the investigation of infertility. Hence the key position of the basal body temperature chart in the process, as mentioned here. (For details of investigations and treatments, see Appendices I–IV.) One clinic is reported as being extraordinarily insensitive to these feelings in instructions for the taking of the temperature on which the chart is based. This is an extreme example, not like the instructions given at the clinic I studied, but it brings into focus the clash of medical and patient expectations which can so complicate their co-operation, particularly in relation to sexual matters.

1. You will shake down the *rectal* thermometer, place it on the bedstand, and set the clock radio for the same time each morning.
2. You should go to bed at the same hour each night.
3. Avoid use of alcohol or smoking if possible.
4. In the morning, when the alarm goes off, the *husband* should gently awaken the wife and insert the rectal thermometer for 5 minutes.
5. When the temperature is taken, they may go back to sleep if they wish.
6. The couple *will* have sexual relations on the nights of days 11, 13, 15, 17 each cycle.
7. Sexual relations at other times may be whatever the *husband* wishes.

(Menning 1977: 127; author's *italics*)

The literature confirms the extent to which the sex life of couples undergoing infertility investigation is affected: sex being made to feel mechanical or pointless and solely for reproduction, not enjoyment. Seastrunk (1984) reported sexual difficulties in 42 per cent of the couples interviewed.

Taken with the findings of the literature in relation to the psychological components of infertility, one must conclude that the effects of this experience on sexual adjustment may be substantial, particularly in the aftermath of diagnosis. There is little evidence, however, of a significantly deleterious effect over the long term, or that sexual problems frequently preceded a diagnosis of infertility, other than amongst those with a non-consummated relationship. It is not a matter of controversy that the experience of infertility and its investigation is, potentially at least, a very distressing experience. Some of this material has already been covered. This section will give more detail of some of the approaches to this experience developed in the literature.

Emotional impact

Discussions of the emotional effects of childlessness acknowledge the distress often experienced. The ideas of psychologists including Erikson

(1950), Bowlby (1969) and C. Murray Parkes (1986), have been influential in the approaches to be found in Menning (1977) and the Houghtons (1977). These ideas will be found reflected in the experiences of childless couples in this study. Menning's model (1977) suggests that reactions to the distress of infertility follow a pattern akin to bereavement:

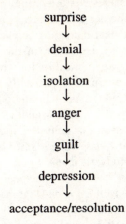

surprise
↓
denial
↓
isolation
↓
anger
↓
guilt
↓
depression
↓
acceptance/resolution

As will be seen, my study suggests that all these reactions are found, although they are not necessarily experienced as a simple, linear process.

Surprise

People assume that they will be able to conceive without difficulty. This is reflected in much that has been written on the subject. This lack of preparedness might be seen as but one aspect of the pronatalist attitudes that affect all our society (see Chapter 3). A couple might well react with surprise, shock, and disbelief at the dawning realisation that conception is not going to occur with the dramatic suddenness that family planning propaganda portrays in alerting the unwary to the dangers of unplanned parenthood. As Menning remarks:

> How ironic for a couple to practise birth control for years and then discover infertility existed all along. How ironic for a couple to question desire or ability to parent and finally make the decision to do it, only to find the decision was not their's to make.
>
> (Menning 1977: 105)

This irony will be an important component in the surprise, and any suspicion that the previous birth control practice might have inhibited the capacity to conceive will exacerbate this reaction. There may be many cases in which there is little surprise, if any, where, for example, the woman had experienced continued gynaecological problems for some time, or the man had sustained a genital injury. As will become clear in this study, the power of assumptions about the universality of fertility may even protect individuals in this situation from anticipating the truth. Erikson (1950) introduces the idea of life stages: maturity requires that certain life tasks are achieved successfully. He writes of generativity as the essential experience of reproduction. The clear and damaging implication of this approach is that it is hardly possible to develop a mature personality without the experience of parenthood – an implication for which there appears to be no evidence in the literature, and none appeared in this study. It also appears to rule out the responsible rejection of parenthood, except in circumstances involving important alternative goals – another striking example of the pronatalist attitudes evident in our culture. Erikson argues that failure to attain generativity leads to a state called 'self-absorption' which involves stagnation and personal impoverishment. In such a situation, the individual becomes absorbed with his or her own personal needs and comforts. The notion of personal impoverishment is one that many infertile people would recognise as relevant to their feelings about their situation, whilst not, perhaps, having the generalised implications of self-absorption and personality stagnation posited by Erikson.

Denial

The stance is that 'this can't be happening to me!' Although it is unlikely to be an available strategy for most infertile couples, there may be situations, such as the one encountered in this study, where it has longer term value for the couple. The practice of encouraging normal intercourse around the time of DI, in the absence of subsequent genetic testing, enables a couple (where sperm count is not zero) to claim that normal conception did occur, denying the male subfertility.

Isolation

This is an aspect of the general presumption of universal fertility already mentioned. Much of the correspondence from new members received by NAC and carried in *Issue* and *NACK* emphasises the isolation experienced by the childless without others in the same position to turn to and discuss their concerns. Another aspect of this involves the diffidence still evident in the discussion of personal problems, particularly in the sexual area. This study reveals the extent of this inhibition and diffidence. The isolation is, partly, the inevitable result of attempts to keep the infertility hidden from others, and thus self-imposed, although nonetheless painful. This might have undesirable consequences in a number of ways: reducing the sources of help available; encouraging misleading notions of why the couple concerned are not having children, perhaps reinforcing negative stereotypes; perhaps permitting untrue ideas to arise concerning the location of the problem (something some women with infertile husbands sometimes actively sought in order to protect the man concerned; cf. Miall 1986).

In a survey of elderly people, Qureshi and Walker (1989) report that, although those having one or two children more often reported feeling lonely than the childless, those without children less often reported any intimate relationships. This perhaps amounts to some suggestion that subjectively, if not objectively, the isolation decreases over time. Bierkens in his survey found that:

> For many couples, childlessness is experienced as emptiness, a sense of not belonging, a deficiency in one's perspective of the future, a lack of purpose in life. In addition there is often the fear of having to rely on strangers in old age, and a fear of severe loneliness upon the loss of the marital partner.
>
> (Bierkens 1975: 180)

The high incidence of suicidal behaviour amongst childless people, particularly the elderly, may be evidence of the isolating impact of childlessness.

Isolation may also have its functional aspect, as Jones (1991) and Menning (1977) point out. It is commonly reported, as emerged in this study, that mixing with parents and children, or child-focused situations, become extremely painful for infertile people. Particularly in the early stages, many people in this position will avoid such situations. Isolation, in this respect, offers emotional protection for those involved; although it is also often reported that the isolation is initiated frequently by those with children (e.g. Pfeffer and Woollett 1983).

Anger

The Robertsons (see Robertson 1953), in their classic studies of the reactions of children to brief separations from their parents, entitled this stage 'protest'. This is also the feeling encapsulated in the title of Stanway's book on infertility, *Why Us?* (1980), the sense that unkind fate has singled the individual out of so many for whom the only fertility problem is preventing conception. This feeling might be exacerbated by the emphasis given in the media and public discussion (as it feels to the infertile at least) to the subjects of contraception and abortion. Two processes might be operating in producing this anger.

An immediate consequence of infertility is the surrender of a sense of control over one's body and important life decisions. The medical profession has to be given access to parts of one's life and behaviour usually regarded as entirely private, engendering a feeling of helplessness. The other aspect of loss of control is the extent to which it is necessary to consider sexual matters when taking decisions which would normally be quite unrelated – e.g. timing of holidays, short separations for work or recreational purposes, etc. Other sorts of decisions might also be affected, such as whether to move house or job, now tied up with access to fertility treatment facilities and changing expectations of family size; pattern of daily activity; recreational pursuits; whether to work or not, and at what sort of occupation.

The second explanation is an extension of the first: personal defence mechanisms operate to protect the individual from the sense of personal failure or betrayal by the partner; these feelings may be projected outwards as anger onto convenient authority figures, in this case doctors, hospitals, family, and friends. In our culture, which discourages the open expression of anger, this is particularly a feature which requires careful attention, if anger which is neither acknowledged nor expressed is not to become an additional source of inter- and intrapersonal distress.

Guilt

The feminist analysis of the sexual politics of women's sickness suggests that common 'first stage' prescriptions for infertility might make the woman feel guilty. Being told to take more rest, not to work or avoid demanding work situations, and being asked to discuss previous contraceptive practices and any abortions are common initial strategies taken by clinics and reflected in lay attitudes. All of these focus on the woman in ways which are likely to make her feel guilty at being unable to conceive. Pfeffer and Woollett (1983) note from their discussions the extent to which such advice is given to the woman even before there is any evidence that it is she who has the fertility problem. This situation, argue Ehrenreich and English (1974), is part of the concept of female invalidism that permeates medical thinking in relation to women: the victim feels that she is to blame.

Infertile people are encouraged to review their histories in the sort of detail which makes it likely that they *will* find something about which to feel guilty. Those without a fertility problem could have identical histories but, without the pressures of fertility investigation, would not be made to feel guilty. Everyone, given the opportunity or pressure for such a review, would find something discreditable. The careful search for a cause which infertility investigation involves may lead to self-blame, as will be seen in this study. These guilt-producing experiences include abortions, contraception, premarital sex, venereal disease, masturbation, divorce, unusual sexual practices.

> Fertile people may experience any and all of these situations and never feel a pang of guilt. The infertile person makes a direct cause-and-effect relationship.

> (Menning 1977: 108)

In ape societies infertile females lose social status (JWPT 1991), so in human society guilt feelings might damage the individual's self-esteem.

Depression

Mahlstedt claims that:

> any one of these losses could precipitate a depressive reaction in an adult . . . Depression, characterised by a sense of hopelessness and despair, is a very common consequence of the diagnosis and treatment of infertility.

> (Mahlstedt 1985)

This may particularly be the case where the infertility is unexplained.

The rates of suicide and attempted suicide are of interest here. Whilst parental status does appear in the literature as one of the variables, studies do not separate out the involuntarily childless from the voluntarily, or those whose children died prematurely or left home prior to the suicide. Therefore, whilst studies find that the childless are over-represented amongst those who attempt or complete suicide (Halbwachs 1930, Stengel 1964), there is no evidence that the experience of infertility *per se* often leads to such behaviour.

Grief

It is this theme that the Houghtons (1977, 1984) took up strongly. They saw this grief as particularly difficult to cope with because there is no object of the grief, rather it is the loss of 'what might have been' and therefore 'unfocused'.

Childlessness may involve various kinds of loss:

- relationship with a child
- status/prestige of being a parent

- self-confidence
- stake in the future
- vicarious fulfilments of parenthood
- healthy self-image
- self-esteem
- security in sickness or old age
- symbolic value of parenthood
- fertility/potence
- experience of pregnancy
- security in the infertile relationship.

The Houghtons (1984) put this succinctly, as the 'three negations':

1. Thwarted love; the love a parent gives to, and receives from, a child.
2. Peripherality; those unable to establish the conventional family feel themselves crucially different, and in that sense somewhat peripheral socially. The increased frequency of alternative family styles is not accepted as softening the experience for the childless, as they are not able to make a choice.
3. Genetic death; the realisation that their genes will not be passed on through countless generations unborn; their death will be final.

Childless couples in this study will speak of their sense of loss and grief.

Acceptance/resolution

Finally should come the stage of acceptance. All the theorists of grief and bereavement see mourning as a healthy process which, properly completed, leads to acceptance and resolution; they also recognise the possibility of blockages occurring. As Menning observes, several factors conspire to inhibit this process. Firstly, the loss may not be recognised by others. Secondly, social attitudes still seem to make the loss in some respects unmentionable, being associated with sexual matters. Thirdly, the loss may not be absolute, in that for so many couples fertility will not be zero, and hope, however remote, might remain until the woman's menopause. Finally, the childless couple may lack strong social support networks which would enable them to deal with the feelings without fear of being left without support. All the literature of people's experiences previously referred to accepts that this process might take a long time to complete, and that, just as with grief, the pain will never go away entirely, but lie hidden to emerge on occasion.

My infertility resides in my heart as an old friend. I do not hear from it for weeks at a time, and then, a moment, a thought, a baby announcement or some such thing, and I will feel the tug – maybe even be sad or shed a few tears. And I think, 'There's my old friend.' It will always be part of me . . .

(Menning 1977: 117)

SUMMARY

Childlessness today is recognised more often than in the past, and more people seek medical help for their predicament, although it is difficult to be certain whether that reflects a real increase in infertility or simply a greater willingness to define it as a medical problem.

Knowledge about the causes of childlessness has been increasing dramatically. The contribution of psychological factors is still very controversial. However, there can be little controversy that childlessness has a substantial impact. This study is the first to examine the experiences of childless people over a period of time.

Autobiographical and fictional literature attests to the pains of infertility. However, information about marital disharmony and failure is inconclusive; it would not at the moment be justified to portray infertility as a proven threat to marriage. The presence of children is as frequently identified in the research as a threat to marriage as is their absence, although the evidence appears to tend towards confirming the lay view that, whilst not preventing marital breakdown, children probably inhibit recourse to divorce as a solution.

The psychological and psychiatric studies available on this subject are generally too weak methodologically to give firm answers to questions about the impact of infertility, just as they are in relation to the psychogenesis of infertility. There appears to be more evidence to support the view that infertility has some temporary impact on the individual's personality and sexual functioning, than that it has a permanent, disabling effect.

Material on the emotional impact of infertility generally confirms that pain and distress is very common, if not universally felt. The relevance of this material will be seen in the echoes which emerge in this study.

3 Pronatalism

In considering the plight of those who are unable to have children, it is essential to place them against the background of social attitudes or norms which shape our desires. It is frequently observed that there are persistent pressures to encourage people to have children: our society is pronatalist. As has been observed elsewhere, it is only possible to understand the experiences of the childless if these pressures are clearly understood.

This chapter will consider these attitudes as they appear to influence the involuntarily childless, and the ways in which they experience their situation. This discussion will be used to place these feelings in their context, and offer some insight into the distress and sense of difference which childless couples will describe in the results of this study. I shall be concerned in particular with the impact of these norms on the married couple. Perceptions of marriage are still almost inextricably interwoven with expectations of child-bearing.

The unmarried woman, it might be argued, has occupied a valued place in society particularly for her unique contribution to the welfare professions. This has, to some extent, insulated her from these pressures. As attitudes to marriage change, and the needs of the economy also, the 'protection' this afforded might alter. Historically, shifts can be seen in this society in attitudes to single women over the last century. When spinsterhood has been inevitable for many women, through the shortage of available husbands in the 1920s and 1930s – which coincided with the growth of the welfare professions like teaching, nursing and social work – the spinster has played an invaluable role. As married women and men have become available for this work, possibly the spinster has been more negatively evaluated.

The question of the biological component of the wish to parent will only be addressed briefly. There can be little doubt that genetics and instinct have a role to play, although the relative importance of such factors is a matter of great controversy.

The term 'pronatalism' gained currency in this connection with the publication of Peck and Senderowitz's *Pronatalism: the Myth of Mom and Apple Pie*, which they define thus:

> Simply and literally pronatalism refers to any attitude or policy that is 'pro-birth', that encourages reproduction, that exalts the role of parenthood.
>
> (Peck and Senderowitz 1974: 2)

The ideas embodied in this term found fertile ground upon which to flourish in the United States of the 1970s and 1980s. They meshed well with the concern of feminists to examine the pressures which kept women at home with reduced life chances as compared with men. They also fitted a characteristic interest of those decades in 'alternative' life styles; for many women the very idea of 'alternatives' was predicated on a radical rethinking of the woman's role as mother. This position is central to the argument of influential books by Adrienne Rich (1977) and Firestone (1972). One result of this interest was the establishment of voluntary organisations devoted to supporting the aspirations of the voluntarily childless against the perceived weight of social opinion. The National Alliance for Optional Parenthood in the United States was followed by the British Organisation of Non-Parents.

> Pronatalism is the attitude that exalts motherhood and assumes or encourages parenthood for all. It is found in nearly all of the institutions in society: churches, schools, advertising, media, law and medicine – and of course families. Pronatalism can be as direct as the question 'When are you going to start your family?' or as subtle as income tax exemptions for children.
>
> (NAOP)

In their influential study of fertility behaviour in Ipswich, Busfield and Paddon (1977) emphasise the importance of the climate of ideas in structuring and supporting reproductive behaviour.

Owens, in discussing the position of childless men, points out that

> in order to understand why people want children we must pay attention to the norms, values and beliefs people hold about them, and about reproduction generally.
>
> (Owens 1982: 74)

This chapter is concerned with the extent to which the prevailing ideology is one that advocates and supports having children, but in popular discussion or in the academic literature, rarely asks the question 'Why have children?'.

PRONATALIST ATTITUDES

Evidence for these attitudes may be seen in much of the literature concerning infertility and childlessness. Philipp and Carruthers (1981: 15) state:

A couple who want a baby are not 'normal' until they get what they want.

Lamson *et al.* (1951) claim that:

what creates unhappiness is not so much the absence of children as the absence of the desire for children.

Miall (1986), in reviewing the literature, argues that:

contemporary endorsement of the fertility norms of having and wanting children transcends sex, age, race, religion, ethnic, and social class divisions in North America.

It has been noted that such attitudes are closely bound up with beliefs about marriage and children. Veevers (1980) claims that mothering and femininity have become synonymous in our society, as represented by four such beliefs:

a. children strengthen marriage and are an indispensible expression of marital love;
b. children are essential to the physical and mental well-being of men and women, particularly women;
c. parenthood is an innately determined need;
d. children confirm masculine and feminine sexual identity and competence.

Material has been presented in Chapter 2 concerning the evidence for some of these beliefs, which in substantial measure was found to be lacking. The debate about a parental, and specifically maternal, instinct was not opened there. This has been the focus for much writing in recent years, which is usefully summarised by Boulton (1983) in her book *On Being a Mother*. Her discussion is noteworthy for its attention to all the competing perspectives on this increasingly emotive subject, rather than for any reiteration of the polemics to be found in literature which rejects any such concept as 'maternal instinct'. There is, however, no argument that the concept has had undoubtedly negative effects for women (e.g. Menning 1977, Dowrick and Grundberg 1980, Eichenbaum and Orbach 1983, Spallone 1989).

Boulton illustrates the way in which biology and ethology might contribute to a broadly based understanding of all the components of parenting behaviour. In reality, regrettably, these perspectives can be, and have been, used to deny the importance of sociological and cultural factors in shaping perceptions of such behaviour.

Dominian, in considering the nature of marital breakdown emphasised:

> Children are one of the main purposes of marriage . . . Couples who have a positive attitude and desire children are clearly more likely to make a successful marriage.
>
> (Dominian 1968: 97)

Despite the significant changes taking place in marriage and the family with the advent of reliable contraception, abortion and divorce and altered perceptions of appropriate roles for women:

> in none of these structural changes do women find support for child-lessness . . . Whatever the reasons for, or causes of, her childlessness the non-mother is still not seen as a proper person.
>
> (Porter 1980: 24)

An article in *New Society* put the effect of these attitudes starkly:

> The childless are seen as selfish, hedonistic, irresponsible and immature. Sterile women are regarded as cold; sterile men as lacking in virility or homosexual. It is doubtful whether even the most enlightened couples remain unaffected by the stigma.
>
> (Laurance 1982)

Baum reports experiences of this constellation of attitudes in relation to the voluntarily childless, where GPs were asked to arrange sterilisation.

> The general attitude they found among medical practitioners was that they ought to have children, and by implication want them, and that even if they did not at the present time, they might in the future.
>
> (Baum 1982)

It should be remembered, however, that such criticism does neglect the numbers of men and women who have sterilisations performed and subsequently seek reversals. The clinician will also be acutely aware of the very real difficulties involved in reversing sterilisation successfully.

It might be concluded from a survey of the literature in demography and sociology that these disciplines are as much imbued with pronatalist assumptions as all others. Anderson (1971) notes the difficulty that sociologists have in standing back to look at family patterns; they tend not to ask why people marry but why they divorce; they ask why people choose to have so many children, rather than why any.

In recent studies, substantially more interest has been shown in voluntary childlessness, viewed from a deviance perspective in particular, than in involuntary childlessness (Veevers *var.*, Miall 1986). Although starting with this view, Porter (1980) was led to conclude that her title 'Willing deviants . . .' was not wholly appropriate in that her respondents appeared not to accept a view of themselves as deviant.

Sara Maitland, one of the contributors to *Why Children?*, reflects the positive attitudes associated with child-bearing thus:

> There was an added bonus which I had not consciously been seeking, but which had probably appealed to some sneaky part of my psyche: I was miraculously restored to my mother's love and approval. I was having a baby: for her that meant I was a good girl and a good woman.
>
> (Dowrick and Grundberg 1980: 83)

Busfield and Paddon argue the position which appears little changed today:

> The misery and disappointment that attaches to childlessness is a common feature of the values surrounding reproduction, and is evidence of the almost universal emphasis on the importance and desirability of becoming a parent.
>
> (Busfield and Paddon 1977)

ORIGINS OF PRONATALISM

Menning claims that:

> From the earliest recordings of mankind there has been an obsession with fertility. Fertility of people and fertility of the land were necessary for survival, and the forces at play were thought to be one and the same.
>
> (Menning 1977: 87)

She goes on to review the potent symbols of mythology in relation to fertility, and the taboos and rituals that are universal in a variety of forms in relation to the processes of reproduction and fertility. Pearl Binder offers a thorough study of fertility symbols in her book *Magic Symbols of the World* (1972). This obsession may be seen as a universal and characteristic feature of all life, much as Darwinian biologists perceive the drive to pass on one's genes to the next generation (cf. Dawkins, *The Selfish Gene*, 1976). It is not uncommon in historical and contemporary non-industrial cultures for the institution of marriage to depend on the proven fertility of the woman. In such cultures marriage was readily terminated if the woman failed to bear a child, and in some cases the marriage was not formalised until the birth of the first child (Tichauer 1963 in Richardson and Guttsmacher 1967).

In most societies failure to bear children has a direct effect on marriage
... In most primitive societies infertility is an occasion for the reduced
status of women at least.

(Mead and Newton 1967)

At certain times in all societies there is likely to be a need for children for their
economic value. Mead and Newton (1967) summarise the importance of
children in pre-industrial societies as being their economic contribution from
an early age in the care of siblings and productive work for the family unit.

The economic status of children is less clear in modern industrial
societies. It has been found that careful economic calculations do not play
a large part in the decision to become pregnant. If they had, family size
would vary directly with disposable income, whereas the consistent evidence of demographers is the reverse. Baum argues that 'in economic
terms, children have become a liability rather than a benefit' (1980: 53).
Becker (1960) writes of their economic status as consumer durables, a
rather extreme view of the wider recognition that children are significant
consumers of wealth, rather than producers, and have a value in our society
for the display of wealth (cf. Owens 1982). This is expressed in a newspaper article as follows:

For economic and political reasons, we must go on having children to
survive. Children create consumer demand; they create work, catering
for their needs, schooling them, feeding them, ensuring that every one
forces its own spending spree.

(McLoughlin 1984)

Studies of family intentions have consistently noted, however, the importance of economic calculations in deciding on the timing and interval of
births (Cartwright 1976, Dunnell 1979).

Poster (1978) notes the continued emphasis our society places on children
as bearers of lineage within the aristocracy; a thesis borne out in the practice of
subjecting the chosen bride of the heir to the throne of Great Britain to
gynaecological examination before announcement of the betrothal; the heir is
not medically examined to assess *his* fertility. This was widely reported on the
engagement in 1981 of Lady Diana Spencer to the Prince of Wales.

Hoffman and Hoffman summarise the non-economic values of children
which are likely to contribute to the pronatalist pressures in society (these
may be compared with the issue of loss discussed in Chapter 2). They
suggest that parenting represents:

- achievement of adult status and social identity;
- expansion of self to a larger entity and the achievement of immortality;
- moral reasons, the opportunity for self-sacrifice and being unselfish;

- emotional security of the family;
- stimulation and fun derived from children;
- opportunities for creativity, accomplishment and competence;
- opportunity for power and influence over children;
- social comparison and competition in them as visible signs of prestige and potence.

(Hoffman and Hoffman 1973)

These values might be regarded both as evidence of pronatalist assumptions, and, to some extent, as reasons for them.

Margaret Mead (1949) points to the almost universal social structures supporting parenthood; a point echoed by Boulton:

Sociology and social anthropology hold that the desire and capacity to look after children are largely socially created.

(Boulton 1983: 16)

The assertions of organised religion offer particularly clear evidence of the social value placed on procreation. It might be argued that all social movements must have primary regard to their expansion and continuance through reproduction. Religions have clear examples in their writings and moral codes to testify to this.

This commitment to parenthood in western society has been attributed to the Judaeo–Christian tradition which sees children as blessings from heaven and barrenness as a curse or punishment. Like leprosy and epilepsy, infertility bears an ancient social stigma.

(Miall 1986)

Christianity is redolent with such emphasis. In the book of Genesis, Adam and Eve are commanded to 'Be fruitful and multiply'. A number of instances in the Bible portray a perception of childlessness as evidence of withdrawal of the favour of God. In finding favour, fertility returned (e.g. the stories of Sarah, Rachel, Hannah and Elizabeth).

When Rachel saw that she bare Jacob no children . . . she said to Jacob, 'Give me children or else I die!' Jacob's anger was kindled against Rachel and he said, 'Am I in the place of God, who has withheld from you the fruit of the womb?' Then she said, 'Here is my maid Bilhah; go in to her, that she may bear upon my knees, and even I may have children through her.'

(Genesis 30: 1–3)

The Roman Catholic Church still maintains a firm position on the importance of procreation not only in its continued opposition to birth control and abortion, but its proscription of homosexuality, masturbation, the practice of donor insemination and *in vitro* fertilisation. This position was reaffirmed in strict and conservative terms by the 'Instruction on Respect for Human Life in its Origins and on the Dignity of Procreation' (Congregation for the Doctrine of the Faith 1987).

The Anglican Book of Common Prayer emphasises the duty of the married couple to have children:

> It was ordained for the increase of mankind according to the will of God, and that children might be brought up in the fear and nurture of the Lord.
> (Solemnization of Matrimony 1928)

Maitland, whose husband is an Anglican priest, puts the commitment thus:

> And for us, with our brand of religious faith, we both believed that heterosexual love meant sacramental marriage, and sacramental marriage meant parenthood.
> (Dowrick and Grundberg 1980)

The links with Judaism are strong, in this as in other doctrinal matters. An orthodox Jew is enjoined to:

- forgo contraception;
- bear at least one son and one daughter;
- not masturbate (avoiding waste of the seed);
- forswear abortion.

Schwartz *et al.* (1980) point out the ways in which these and other rabbinical laws can seriously inhibit the treatment of infertility. Within the same tradition, Mormonism and Fundamentalist Christianity exert great pressure on their adherents to have children:

> Our prophets tell us that 'no other success can compensate for failure in the home'. Children are desired above wealth, position, degrees or power. 'Families are forever.' 'Our children are our jewels in the crown of eternal life.' . . . Feelings such as these saturate the Utah atmosphere. Perhaps this emphasis is not so great in other geographical areas of the church. But here in Utah, the cultural pressure for raising large, happy families is mind-boggling.
> (Probst 1982)

> One of the things that really caused me so much pain was that as a woman in the fundamentalist community, I was taught I had no rights, just one basic purpose – wife and mother.
> (Smith 1981)

The other great world religions, Islam, Hinduism and Buddhism, all embody prescriptions to encourage child-bearing amongst the faithful. These merit equal attention in our multi-cultural society. I have highlighted the factors in the Judaeo–Christian tradition, as it is those in particular that underpin western medicine.

Pronatalism is firmly grounded in fundamental aspects of our social organisation. It is to be expected that it, therefore, holds considerable influence over us all, particularly those who appear unable or perhaps unwilling to conform.

EVIDENCE OF PRONATALISM

The effects of pronatalism may be seen in many of the institutions and processes of society. In addition, the literature offers evidence of its existence and impact in psychological theories and empirical studies.

Social institutions

Peck and Senderowitz (1974) document in detail the pervasiveness of pronatalist imagery and attitudes in western society. Noting this feature is not unique to this period of history. The same concerns were identified at earlier periods of feminist activity. In 1916 Leta S. Hollingworth wrote in the *American Journal of Sociology*:

> The fact is that child-bearing is in many respects analogous to the work of soldiers: it is necessary for tribal or national existence; it means great sacrifice of personal advantage; it involves danger and suffering, and in a certain percentage of cases, the actual loss of life. Thus we should accept that there would be a continuous social effort to insure the group interest in respect of the population, just as there is a continuous social effort to insure the defense of the nation in time of war. It is clear, indeed, that the social devices employed to get children born, and that get soldiers slain, are in many respects similar.
>
> (Quoted in Peck and Senderowitz 1974)

A NAOP pamphlet 'Pronatalism' (1979) succinctly discusses the areas of social life in which these effects might be seen. The Madonna image is a pervasive and very ancient image in art, not confined to the Christian religion. Some of the earliest art objects known, of the Upper Palaeolithic period dating from perhaps 35 millennia before Christ, appear to be fertility charms (e.g. the Venus of Willendorf, described in Bazin 1958). The importance of the phallus as a religious image is also as old as organised religion itself; from Sumerian cults to the lingam of modern Hinduism or the soaring spires of Christianity.

The advertising industry uses the family and parenthood intensively to support commercial trade in everything from gravy powder to motor cars and from washing powder to railways. It has often been observed that it is hard to know whether it is the product or the value of parenthood that is receiving the hardest sell. Any cursory examination of the mass media and entertainment will reveal many examples of the high status accorded to parenthood, and the tendency to glamorise and romanticise families with children.

The political process always demonstrates, to some extent, a concern with policies which promote parenthood. Particular social conditions, and the perception of them, will dictate the extent to which this concern is explicit. Baum (1980) produced an interesting analysis of the frequency with which the family was mentioned in the election manifestos of the three principal British political parties this century. The elections of 1945 and 1950 and again those from 1966 on showed very substantially increased rates of reference to the family; these might be said to be times when the family was seen to be under threat. More explicit pronatalist policies may be seen in Stalin's motherhood medals, and continuing state-sanctioned religious opposition to contraception and abortion in, for example, Argentina and Ireland.

> Every woman of child-bearing age in Romania is being questioned about her sex life in an unprecedented drive to increase the country's birth rate. President Nicolae Ceausescu wants a minimum of four children per family. Women with ten children will be awarded the Heroic Mother's medal. Childless couples will be fined.
>
> (*Issue*, Winter 1987)

It will be of interest to see whether the demise of Ceausescu will see changes in these policies. The same policies are seen in more subtle form in the taxation and social security laws in operation in all western nations, which universally favour parents over non-parents in subsidising the costs of children. There are certainly contemporary policies which pull in the opposite direction, particularly in Third World concern for the effects of over-population on their hard-pressed economies. However, the fates of Sanjay Gandhi and the Congress Party in India in the early 1980s are testimony to the difficulty such policies face. Even the totalitarian government of the People's Republic of China has experienced severe difficulties in promoting the one-child family policy, and has been forced to backtrack.

It is not an overstatement that society typically creates many institutions to support its continuance in the breeding and raising of children.

Psychoanalytic theories

The impact of these approaches to understanding the nature of childlessness is outlined within the discussion of the causes of infertility and in relation to its psychological and emotional impact (Chapter 2). Chertok (1969) provides a useful summary of the implications of these perspectives for motherhood and childbirth. Feminist literature often points out the inherent sexism of some of the fundamental tenets of Freudian theory, particularly the concepts of penis envy and the Oedipus complex (cf. Oakley 1981).

> Psychoanalytic theory, then, implies that motherliness is a normal char-
> acteristic of a mature woman's femininity; that 'motherliness in action'
> is naturally rewarding; and consequently that the experience of
> dissatisfaction in motherhood is evidence of developmental problems in
> a woman and poor adjustment to her feminine psychosexual identity.
>
> (Boulton 1983: 3)

Deutsch, in her influential work *The Psychology of Women* (1945), clearly equates womanhood with motherhood. In the developmental psychology which arose from psychoanalysis, pioneered by Erikson (1950), there runs a consistent thread which perceives the achievement of motherhood, and to a lesser extent fatherhood, as a necessary step in growth to maturity and full independence as a person. Erikson labels one of the vital stages 'gener-ativity' (see Chapter 2). It is interesting to see the way in which feminist psychotherapy is attempting to come to terms with psychoanalytic concepts. Thus the gender-biased language of Erikson is transformed by Eichenbaum and Orbach:

> When two people want to have a child together they are making a
> statement about their feelings for one another. A child represents the
> merger and intimacy of the couple relationship . . . Achieving love and
> intimacy has a sense of movement forward, a working towards some-
> thing, creating something together, working towards and believing in a
> future . . . The birth of a child represents this move forward and the
> belief in life and growth.
>
> (Eichenbaum and Orbach 1983: 136)

There are still clear signs of a shared conception that full realisation of personal potential is bound up with the achievement of parenthood.

Successful mastering of the past is a prerequisite for women's psychic health; otherwise new situations provoke new traumas . . . The reproductive experience gives woman the opportunity to master old anxieties by mastering new ones.

(Deutsch 1945: 49–50)

Although the influence of psychoanalytic concepts has never been as strong in the psychology or psychiatry of the UK as it has been in other parts of the western world, notably the United States, they have still had a profound impact on the way we view our personal and social lives. The fascinating confluence of radical social critiques and psychoanalytic views of individual mental function which may be observed at the moment will surely delay the nemesis so confidently predicted by Eysenck (1986).

Empirical evidence

There has been an explosion of interest in recent years in the sociology of the family, fuelled by feminist critiques of traditional patterns of family life. Contained therein are data concerning the experience of pronatalism which may be considered briefly.

Blood and Wolfe found substantial evidence for these pressures: 26 per cent thought of children as the most valuable part of marriage, and 28 per cent as the second most valuable. Given their choice over again, only 3 per cent would not have had children; and 36 per cent replied that there was nothing good about childlessness. Only one person in 599 interviewed felt there was nothing good about children. The picture they built up was one of substantial normative support for child-bearing.

> Most childless wives clearly believe having children would be worth any disadvantage.

(Blood and Wolfe 1955)

Dr Rajkumar of the International Planned Parenthood Foundation at a BON (British Organisation of Non-Parents) meeting claimed that, despite the very considerable hazards of childbirth in the Third World, there was no evidence that the availability of contraception was increasing the popularity of childlessness, rather that it was being used to bring the preferred and actual family size more closely together (Rajkumar 1982).

Owens, in looking at the experience of childless husbands, states:

> Childlessness was negatively valued. Those who wished to be childless were stigmatised as selfish, while those who were unable to have children were pitied.

(Owens 1982: 75)

Baum (1980) and Porter (1980) have interesting observations to make on the experience of social pressure felt by their voluntarily childless respondents. Unlike the consistent conclusions of North American researchers (e.g. Pohlman 1969, Houseknecht 1979, Veevers 1980, Miall 1986) they reported that the childless did *not* experience continuous, oppressive social pressure to the same extent. Porter notes that:

> There appeared to be a moral imperative that the married will want children, whether or not they can and do choose to have them, and that not wanting them or wanting other things more was likely to result in accusations of selfishness and immaturity.

> (Porter 1980: 324)

However, she goes on to admit that her respondents, whilst apparently feeling fairly aware of it, failed to document clear instances of pronatalist pressure. Unlike Cooper *et al.* (1978) who disparagingly label this perception 'pseudo-paranoia', Porter is not inclined to reject the reality of this pressure so easily. She inclines to the view that this finding reflects, in part at least, a disinclination to discuss these feelings rather than their being an illusion. She observed a peak in these perceived feelings around the fourth year of marriage, which subsequently tapered off. Porter also claims that the pressure was unduly placed on the woman; although her sample contained very few male respondents. This finding was supported by this study and Connolly *et al.* (1987). The literature suggests that the significant distinction may be that many childless people feel under social pressure to have children, but not stigmatised by their failure to do so.

SUMMARY: WHY HAVE CHILDREN?

The title of Dowrick and Grundberg's book *Why Children*? was intended to be provocative. It emphasises the extent to which this question is so rarely asked, not just by the ordinary person but also by the academic. They make this plain in their introduction to the accounts given by individual women for taking such a major step, particularly the well-educated, middle-class, feminist, career-oriented women they invited to contribute, and to whom the book is clearly addressed. Previous sections have considered some of the possible answers to this question.

> Our aim was to convey the complexity, the deep personal significance of the decision whether or not to have children, the most irrevocable and important one that most of us will make.

> (Dowrick and Grundberg 1980: 8)

Wordsworth expresses the positive qualities of this inevitability thus:

. . . a child, more than all other gifts,

That earth can offer to declining man,
Brings hope with it, and forward-looking thoughts.

('Michael', lines 154–6, Wordsworth 1984)

In his recent autobiography, one of Britain's most distinguished living natural scientists, Sir Alan Parkes, gives his views on this matter.

> The reasons why people want a family would make a fascinating study. Very few, I imagine, would honestly say that they do so because they are sure that their offspring will be glad to have been born. What the children think about it all is not usually considered very carefully . . . We come thus to the curious paradox that parents may make great efforts and prolonged sacrifices for children produced for essentially egotistical motives.

(Parkes 1985: 417)

He goes on to show remarkably little insight into the depth of feeling of those who are unable to make the choice freely.

> If we accept that individuals have a right to reproduce, if only to a limited extent, have those who are unable to do so the right to be assisted? My own view is that, since there is no lack of fertile people, they should accept their disability and direct their creative urges else-where . . . However, most people, including the medical profession as a whole, think otherwise.

(Parkes 1985: 424)

This statement echoes the extreme rationalism that appears to pervade some commentary on this matter.

> 'Family intentions' surveys have concentrated on how many children of what sex couples want, on the extent to which families are truly planned and on whether so-called 'family planning' services help or hinder them to match precept and practice.

(Oakley 1981: 225)

The evidence tends to support the earlier view expressed by Macintyre (1976) and Payne (1978): not only do researchers not address this question, but neither do couples in making their fertility decisions.

The first survey to acknowledge in its questions the possibility that married couples might not want any children was that of Peel and Carr (1975). They found only 4 per cent of the couples interviewed were of this view. In asking their respondents what choice they would make about children if starting again, Blood and Wolfe (1955) found 3 per cent in

Detroit and 1 per cent in Michigan who said 'none'. This difference between urban and rural respondents is consistently reported in North American studies of voluntarily childless people. In answering the question posed in his title 'Is zero preferred?', Blake (1979) gives an unequivocal negative for the great majority of those interviewed. In a comparative survey of family intentions in Europe, it is stated that in no country did the option 'no children' exceed 0.5 per cent as the ideal family size (United Nations 1976).

Busfield and Paddon (1977), Oakley (1979) and Owens (1982) confirm the extent to which, for nearly everyone, the concept of family *ipso facto* requires children.

Work in the United States in particular has attempted to create a model of fertility decision making which suggests a considerable degree of intentionality and rational calculation in the process (see, for example, Shedlin and Hollerbach 1978). Payne's study of the attitudes of couples of child-bearing age to the possibility of having children demonstrates the lack of such a sophisticated calculus.

> For all respondents children were seen to a large extent as the way of demonstrating ordinariness.
>
> (Payne 1978)

Busfield and Paddon (1977) confirmed the extent to which reproductive ideologies are largely about claims to full citizenship and ordinariness; the expected and inevitable outcome of a satisfactory marriage; the membership card for what Rony Robinson (1982) calls 'the freemasonry of the fertile'. The close association between marriage and childbirth is frequently reported, and has already been referred to as one of the contributory pressures to have children. Cartwright (1976) notes the prevalence of pregnancy as the precipitant of marriage. Thornes and Collard (1979) note the frequent response giving children as the primary motive for marriage instead of co-habitation. This is not to deny that there are those for whom this is a 'dichotomous choice' (Veevers 1979), and one that may be being made in favour of childlessness with increasing frequency. These writers would accept that, for the great majority, the weight of evidence is that there is no choice to be made, 'it's natural' (Owens 1982). It may be the case, as Burgoyne (1987) argues, that as unmarried co-habitation becomes more popular, the pressure on the married to have children might be increasing.

Oakley, in her exploration of this 'decision', notes:

> People do not have clear motives so far as having children is concerned: few organise their lives according to some overall plan. The subject of

children provokes ambivalent feelings, so that 'planning' is a euphemism for allowing one particular feeling or pressure to gain an upper hand . . . Despite its complexity, the question 'did you want or plan a baby?' may be easier to answer than the parallel question 'why did you want a baby?'. This taps a minefield of half explored motives and reasons.

(Oakley 1979: 32–3)

In conclusion, it is not to be wondered at that those who are unable to fulfil the injunction to have children should frequently experience their social position as isolated and painful. There is a great weight of normative pressure to choose and attain the role of parent. It would not be possible to understand fully the situation of the involuntarily childless without taking full account of the cultural, social and moral climate within which their wishes and attitudes are formed.

4 Childlessness in community and clinic

Some interesting features emerged in the surveys upon which this book is based. In certain respects the couples attending the Infertility Clinic appeared not to be fully representative of the population at large. In comparing the experience of the Clinic study group with the results of the survey of general practitioners (FPS) and the survey of the group general practice (GPS), some of the reasons for these differences will become apparent.

Not all those with a medical problem will seek medical help. The group general practice surveyed served a predominantly working-class area. The lower socio-economic groups are those that many studies have noted as least likely to be well served by health care.

A fundamental question of the sociology of medicine is stated by Mechanic and Volkart (1961) thus:

> Two persons having the same symptoms, clinically considered, may behave quite differently; one may become concerned and immediately seek medical aid, while the other may ignore the symptoms and not consider seeking treatment at all.

Last (1963) coined the term 'illness iceberg' to describe this latter group of people. Reeder *et al.* (1978) suggest that the close network ties found in working-class communities are particularly associated with a protracted period of 'lay referral' (i.e. discussion with lay members of the community expected to know about such things) and thus delayed seeking help from the formal medical system. The GPS offers some indications of the extent of under-referral occurring in a working-class community; the numbers of hidden childless.

Zola's classic paper 'Pathways to the doctor: from person to patient' (1973) notes that the timing of the decision to seek medical help cannot be understood with reference to the symptoms alone, but, he argues, is 'based on a break in the accommodation to the symptoms'. The Clinic study will offer some information on the nature of this break as experienced by infertile couples.

Another important determining factor appears to be that of gender. Ehrenreich and English (1974) and Oakley (1984) ruefully note the extent to which women's problems have become medicalised. Many studies have noted marked differences in the rate at which women and men seek medical help. Scambler and Scambler (1984) suggest that the reproductive process is clearly one important factor in this differential usage, but that there may also be important differences in such matters as interest in and concern with health which are related to gender bias during socialisation. During 1987, the average number of consultations with a GP was four for men and six for women: 13 per cent of the men and 18 per cent of the women had consulted their GP in the previous 14 days (OPCS 1989). The Clinic study will draw attention to the greater burden imposed on the women during infertility investigation.

THE HIDDEN CHILDLESS

It is difficult to determine the relative sizes of voluntarily and involuntarily childless groups in the community, as well as the prevalence of child-lessness itself.

As defined in Chapter 1, the GPS produced a figure of 1,166 ever-married or co-habiting women over the age of 16, of whom 197 (16.9 per cent) were childless; i.e. had given birth to no live children, but were neither using contraception nor sterilised. Twenty-five couples (2.1 per cent) were childfree or were delaying children, in that they were currently using contraception or one or both partners had been sterilised. (In future the three groups, as explained in Chapter 1, will for simplicity be described as childless, childfree or parous. The characteristics to which these groups refer will be described collectively as 'childedness'.) This rate of 16.9 per cent or 1:6 is somewhat larger than some other estimates, and may in part reflect the predominantly working-class character of this area, unlike the referrals to the Infertility Clinic.

The analysis for the purposes of this study concentrated on identifying a childless group for further contact and comparing the childless women, as already defined, on various parameters with those who appeared to be childfree and parous. Conclusions from this analysis must be tentative, particularly in view of the bias towards higher social class, older and female patients observed when comparing those who responded to the survey and those who did not. However, the patients who did respond to the survey were broadly representative of the population of the practice area, when compared with the results of the Census 1981 using the SASPAC computer package. (Detailed analysis of the GPS may be found in Monach 1987.) These results should therefore be seen as pointers of interest for further research.

Age

There was a strong association between childedness and age. Sixty-five per cent of the childless were 65 or over, but only 39.1 per cent of the parous women. This would be expected for two reasons. Firstly, reproductive medicine has developed out of all recognition since 1945: when many of these pensioners were at the peak of their child-bearing years, modern treatments were not available. Secondly, it is likely that during those years women were much less likely to have sought advice if they did not conceive as they had hoped. This reluctance, we might suppose, would have three sources: a realistic assessment of the limited strategies open to medicine; the cost of medical treatment in the days before the National Health Service for these predominantly working-class patients; a greater diffidence in those days in discussing matters related to sex.

If the results are considered controlling for the effects of the age differences between the groups, taking just those who are past child-bearing age, and therefore of completed fecundity, then the childless group becomes 20.2 per cent of all women ever married, and the childfree still a mere 1.5 per cent. The ratio of 1:5 married women being childless is even larger than common estimates, and perhaps gives support to the view that childlessness is unevenly distributed in the population, being more prevalent in working-class, urban populations than in other parts of the community.

Social class

The association between class and childedness attained clear statistical significance (χ^2 =15.24, *P*=0.0184), although the homogeneity of the patient population meant that the higher social classes were very small, influencing the reliability of the statistical test.

The clearest difference is in the proportion of childless people in the different classes. Whilst only 8.9 per cent in RG class II were childless, 16.9 per cent of RG class III were in that position. Although there has only been speculation that involuntary childlessness is correlated with social class, this evidence appears to support the idea that its prevalence may increase amongst lower social classes. As suggested also by the Black Report (Black 1980), the issues of relative access might repay further investigation. Although evidence concerning those factors inimical to fertility is still relatively undeveloped, it would be fair to say that, so far as environmental factors are concerned, there are class-linked factors which lead in both directions, e.g. contraceptive practice, abortion, industrial hazards, tobacco and drug usage, age of family building. These were more fully considered in relation to the incidence of infertility.

The distribution of those who are childfree is even more sharply defined by class; none of the unskilled manual workers belongs to this group. This would seem to confirm the consistent finding of studies discussed elsewhere that being childfree and delaying family building are both strongly, positively correlated with high social class.

Employment

Substantially fewer childless women were in employment than those who had children, and proportionately more were retired.

It is perhaps surprising to find that the childless without the responsibilities of parenting were less likely to be employed than mothers. The childfree have the expected high rate of employment participation. It might be speculated from this result that the folk wisdom which commonly suggests that stopping work is an important aid to conception might lead to childless women leaving the job market and not returning. They might, therefore, not be taking a full part in the dramatic rise in the rates of women's participation in the economy that has been such a key feature of recent social trends. In 1961 just under 30 per cent of married women were economically active, compared with 49 per cent in 1981 (OPCS 1983). The penalties of childlessness from this evidence might include reduced chances in the labour market compared with those enjoyed by other women. This is rather at odds with the popular stereotype reported by some of the Clinic patients interviewed of the childless as materially better off through the 'selfish' pursuit of career instead of parenthood.

Marriage

There were clear differences between the groups concerning their marital status. This survey (GPS) illustrates the extent to which, in a city working-class community, at least, marriage and childbirth are so much seen as part of the same equation. Of the ever-married women who had children, 43 per cent conceived their first before marriage. The General Household Survey (1983) notes a comparable figure of 22 per cent. This appears to bear out the contention of the doctors in this practice that it was the norm in that community for marriage to be undertaken as the consequence of pregnancy, rather than in preparation for it. In this community failure to conceive during premarital intercourse *may* carry consequences for the woman's chances of marriage.

Although the numbers are very small compared to the total sample, there was little evidence of substantially higher rates of separation and divorce amongst the childless (13 per cent) than amongst the parous (10.3 per cent), even though the childless women, being older, had been married much longer than those with children.

Fertility in women is known to decline with age after the age of 30. As discussed elsewhere, the timing of this decline is not exact and is subject to substantial individual variation. The age of marriage may play an important part in the fertility chances of individual women for this reason. It would be expected, therefore, that the childless women may on the whole have married later than their parous sisters. This proved to be the case in this survey.

Analysis indicates a significant association between increasing age at marriage and the likelihood of being childless, both considering the current marriage ($\chi^2 = 59.0$, $P = 0.0000$) and in considering the first marriage ($\chi^2 = 128.1$, $P = 0.0000$). Cross-tabulating age at current marriage with childedness shows that the childless married consistently later than the parous: 11.2 per cent of the childless married under the age of 19, but 25.6 per cent of the parous. The childless overtake the parous only after the age of 25: 9.3 per cent of these childless women were not married until after the age of 45, at which time nearly all women have become infertile. The same is also true when age at first marriage is cross-tabulated with childedness. Just 13 per cent of the childless were under 19 at this first marriage, compared with 29.9 per cent of the parous; 26.1 per cent of the childless married after the age of 30, but only 4 per cent of the parous.

The childfree married earlier than either of the other groups, confirming the view noted already that most of these women were delaying having children rather than intending not to have any.

The evidence presented here supports the view that one of the most important factors in explaining the rate of childlessness in a community is the age at which women marry. Significant differences were found in comparing the childless women with those who were delaying having children or had decided not to have any, and those who had given birth to children.

Childfree women had been married for a much shorter time than either of the other groups (52.6 per cent less than five years), whereas only 9.1 per cent of the childless and 7.9 per cent of the parous were in this position. This could be taken as further evidence that most of these women were simply delaying their first child rather than having a fixed intention not to have any children. This matches the views of Baum (1980) that for most of her voluntarily childless people it was more appropriate to say they had not (?yet) decided to have children, rather than that they had decided not to have them.

The age distribution of the childfree in this survey would seem to support the view that voluntary childlessness is still an unpopular option amongst the urban working class, whatever the popularity it might be gaining amongst the YUPpies (Young Upwardly-mobile) and DINKs (Double Income No Kids) (Reisz 1987), from whence both Porter (1980) and Baum (1980) drew their respondents.

Religion

In terms of religion, the patient population of this practice was very homogeneous; only 6.1 per cent of the population claimed a religious belief that might have conflicted with the investigation of infertility, nearly all Roman Catholic. There was no significant association with childedness. As discussed in Chapter 3, this might be an important factor in other populations, and in the usage of specialist medical facilities.

Medical history

The survey collected information on what the respondents *themselves* felt to have been serious illness, which must be open to substantial variation; however, as a measure of the individual's sense of well-being, it is of interest.

Perhaps the striking thing is that 57.2 per cent of those replying recorded no serious illnesses. The numbers of illnesses reported were too small for useful attempts at comparing the experience of the childless, childfree and parous women with respect to individual complaints.

The groups could, however, be helpfully compared on the number of illnesses reported (up to the maximum of 'four or more' offered in the questionnaire used). This suggested that the childless are less likely to report serious illness than those with children ($\chi^2 = 19.82$, $P = 0.0110$). Illnesses of the puerperium were so rarely reported that they could not account for the difference in total morbidity. It might, however, be the case that those without children are indeed more healthy, in the way demonstrated in some studies which have considered the impact of children on women and marriages which were reviewed in Chapter 2.

A similar picture is seen on considering the answers about surgical operations experienced. Arguably, the answers to this question are less open to individual idiosyncrasy, requiring no judgement about seriousness, and there being little doubt in the lay mind of what might be regarded as an operation. Memory might be less unreliable in this matter since operations are significant events for most people.

The childless reported significantly fewer operations than the parous or childfree ($\chi^2 = 16.08$, $P = 0.0413$), which the hazards of pregnancy do not appear to explain. As with illness, age is likely to be an important factor in this result; unfortunately, controlling for age reduces the size of the groups to a point where tests are unreliable.

This finding could also be said to contradict the stereotype of the childless woman already mentioned. Self-absorption and limited interests might have been expected to increase the incidence of reported illness, and possibly even the experience of operations. It also seems to suggest improved health amongst childless women. There was no apparent effect of operations related to infertility, of which very few were reported.

The picture presented in this evidence is, perhaps, the surprising one that childless women see themselves, on the whole, as more healthy than their parous sisters. This seems to contradict images of the self-centred childless woman who might be expected to seek more medical attention of all kinds.

Social habits

Surveys of smoking and drinking are notorious for not being answered honestly. However, the consumption rates obtained in this survey were slightly higher than comparable figures from *Social Trends* (matched for age and social class), suggesting that they are at least as reliable, if it is assumed that people under-report.

The proportion of women who reported smoking was 39 per cent (compared with 33 per cent for this social group – CSO 1986). Smoking was significantly less common amongst the childless ($\chi^2 = 19.5$, $P = 0.0034$) than those with children or childfree.

Drinking alcohol showed a similar pattern: 51.4 per cent in this survey compared with 55 per cent of women in the population (CSO 1986) claimed to drink 'occasionally', 'socially', 'for medicinal reasons' or not at all. As with smoking, childless ever-married women were significantly less likely to drink alcohol ($\chi^2 = 28.4$, $P = 0.0004$).

In this survey, the consumption of alcohol or tobacco does not occur more frequently amongst the childless than amongst other ever-married women in the community, as might have been predicted if either were significantly related to the incidence of infertility.

CHILDLESS WOMEN IN THE PRACTICE

As with virtually all medical conditions, not all those who have impaired fertility will find their way to a specialist clinic. Some will accept the failure to conceive as one of those 'quirks' of nature. Either through lack of sufficient determination to have children, or through reluctance to discuss the problem with outsiders in general or doctors in particular, they may take no action to remedy their infertility. There has as yet, as discussed in Chapter 2, been no proper epidemiological study of infertility in this country which could describe the dimensions of the problem and the extent of 'filtering' that is going on.

The General Practice Study offered a population to follow up which could produce some indications for further investigation. The GPS questionnaires, which suggested that the woman concerned was childless – whether childless or childfree in the terms used in the analysis – were extracted. This gave a subsample of 222 women, 197 or 16.9 per cent childless and 25 or 2.1 per cent childfree. Only those under the age of 45 were selected for further contact, it being felt that older women would be too remote from the experiences concerned and might be particularly distressed to have the subject brought up. To these were added two others known to the doctors to be trying without success to conceive a child. This produced a sample of 51 women. For various reasons, including my un-availability and the reluctance of the doctors to implement the previously agreed second-stage survey of those who appeared to be childless, there was a three-and-a-half-year interval before the status of these 51 women was re-examined. Information was obtained from a second questionnaire in 13 cases, and from the doctors and/or medical notes in 34 cases; in four cases the woman had left the practice list and no further information could be obtained.

The results summarised in Table 4.1 suggest that, over a period of three-and-a-half years, a third of those apparently involuntarily childless women had children, only one in 16 seemed to have decided to remain childfree, one in five remained childless but had since ceased to live in a partnership which might have led to her becoming pregnant through separation, widowhood or divorce, and three in ten remained involuntarily childless.

Table 4.1 Childless respondents of subsample

	No.	*%*
Involuntarily childless	16	31.4
No current partner	10	19.6
Now had own children	18	35.4
No information	4	7.8
Childfree	3	5.8
Total	51	100.0

The involuntary childlessness identified by the GPS encompasses a variety of situations, including:

- genetic contraindications to pregnancy
- emotional/psychiatric problems
- recurrent miscarriage
- identified subfertility problems
- family planning identified fertility problem
- failure to conceive, no reason known.

It was striking that of the 16 women who remained childless over this period of at least four-and-a-half years (they were only identified as childless at the first stage if they had failed to conceive for a period in excess of one year), only five requested, and were referred on to, specialist investigation. The indications of this survey are, therefore, that for every three women who fail to conceive a child, only one will seek and receive specialist evaluation of her difficulties. This finding should be treated with caution, in view of the limited numbers of women involved and the nature of the population sampled; however, it does suggest that there is a very substantial amount of uninvestigated involuntary childlessness, perhaps to be found disproportionately in working-class communities such as that studied here.

In the circumstances outlined above, the description 'childfree' is particularly awkward and tentative. On the basis of the limited information available, only one of the three women seemed to fit this category as someone who, in otherwise good health, had chosen not to have children without any reason to think she could or should not do so. The other two fitted that category hypothesised earlier: those women who delay childbirth for various reasons, but then find other difficulties in the way of childbirth which seem to make them decide not to attempt pregnancy. These are the sorts of instances previously referred to which make any attempt to declare a firm distinction between those who are voluntarily childless and those who are involuntarily childless highly problematic. In contrast to the impression given by some North American studies, those who consciously, at an early stage in their reproductive careers, decide they do not want children are probably a very small group of those who might still claim to have chosen to be childless.

The comments made by four of the women who wanted children, and had been (or were being) investigated or treated without success, speak of their experience (quoted verbatim with original spelling from the returned questionnaire):

Whilst our own practitioner has been very understanding and referred us to the hospital specialist, we were told there's nothing wrong with us –

full stop! Then due to myself having a cervical smear test I was referred back to the (A. Hospital) which in turn lead me to being referred to (B. Hospital) due to my infertility since which I have waited one year for an appointment then just as the date was getting near I received a letter this week back dating the appointment a further year. Obviously the experience of wanting a child all these years (12) has not been good and at times upsetting – it would appear that unless you've got money then you simply get forgotten. Both myself and my husband wanted children in our teens, we are now in our 30's, at this rate we'll be in retirement before we even see the specialist.

Had all the tests at (C. Hospital) and (B. Hospital) over a period of 5 years 1972–78. Was obsessed with wanting a child all through that time. Every month's period was a disappointment, found some hospital staff did not understand.

I've been under (B. Hospital) 8 years. First I had fertility drugs, and then artificial insemination, then they new my tubes was blockt, they was going to do them, but I got warts in my vagina from my first husband, that was a big operation, 2 yrs ago. Id got a abcass in my right tube wich made me very ill. *I was very upset looking forward to them clearing my tubes to have a baby to my husband* But this yr. Dr. B at B. Hospital said they couldent do them know. Because the abcess had been to near my tubes. My womb is very healthy, But the only way is *Test tube Baby* I'M on DHSS I havent got the money wich I dont think its fare. My mother has had 10 children and all of them have children twins ect. But that saden me Because Im the only wote hasent had them, I dident want to be left alone if enythink happend to my husband. Im 39 Id been under (B. Hospital) since I was 30. Nearly 9 yrs under (B. Hospital) seamed a waist of time regarding children.

I have found my situation very depressing and very hard to cope with. But at the moment I still feel hopeful.

This survey has produced the finding that for every woman in an urban working-class community who is concerned that she is not producing the child she wants, and is referred for specialist investigation, there may be two who do not seek referral, and therefore remain childless although there might be a remedy. This situation is a matter for concern as it suggests that a considerable proportion of potential patients are not willing to come forward for the available help. As publicity and media attention grow in respect of these problems, it could lead to a substantial increase in the demand which would not be anticipated on the basis of past experience. Without knowledge of the reasons the patients concerned did not choose to be referred for investigation, it is impossible to know accurately the implications of this finding.

The 'hidden childless' seem to be a not inconsiderable number of people, about whom we know very little.

INFERTILITY CLINIC

Tables 4.2 and 4.3 summarise occupation, age, diagnosis and outcome for each of the couples who took part in the study. (The names are, of course, fictitious, and some occupations are disguised.)

The ways in which the study group of 30 couples was recruited were discussed in Chapter 1. This group appeared to be representative of all the patients attending this Clinic, insofar as the limited socio-demographic information recorded in the medical notes permitted comparison.

Connolly *et al.* (1987), surveying 843 couples referred to the same Clinic over ten years, unfortunately only report socio-economic class for comparison with these results. Simple observation in the course of spending almost a year in the Clinic, as well as the comments of staff members, did, however, suggest that this group was fairly typical. It did not entirely match the description offered by one staff member – already quoted in Chapter 1 – although this indicated a clear trend in the social characteristics of the patients.

Socio-demographic features

Early referral for the investigation of infertility is important in view of the decline of fertility with *age*; marked after 35 for women, and after 40 for men (see Stanway 1984, Hull *et al.* 1985, Howe *et al.* 1985). The mean age of the women was 28 years (range 20 to 37) and of the men 29 years (range 21 to 40). The mean age of first legitimate birth at the time was 25.4 years (OPCS 1986b). Taken with the information on the period for which they were unsuccessfully trying for children, this suggests that this group were later than might be expected in their family-building behaviour.

All the couples, except the Holts and Flowers, were *married* when referred to the Clinic. The Holts remained unmarried, which was one of the reasons later advanced for removing their names from the IVF waiting list. The Flowers married during the study. All presented themselves as if married; hence the use of the conventional styles 'husband' and 'wife' throughout this study.

Table 4.2 Key characteristics: women

	Age	Occupation	Diagnosis	Outcome
Coleman	24	Bank clerk	NAD	Px
Carver	32	Secretary	NAD	DI
Ivy	23	Hairdresser	Anovulatory	P
Dorairaj	36	Accounts clerk	Anovulatory	C
Green	26	Cashier	Asynch., endo., adhesions	C
Underwood	32	Secretary	NAD	C
Turner	26	Domestic	Anovulatory	C
Truswell	26	Supervisor	NAD	C
Young	30	Shop assistant	NAD	C
Thurston	22	Packer	Hydrosalpinx, adhesions	Adop.
Grindrod	32	Housewife	Blocked tubes, fibroids	C
Monk	31	Bank clerk	Anovulatory	P
Kitchen	37	Cleaner	Endo., FSH problem	C
Butler	36	Administrator	NAD	Px
Carter	23	Teacher	Anovulatory	(C)
Urmston	32	Travel clerk	Oligomenorrhoea	P
Keith	29	Clerical officer	Endo.,? ovulation problem	P
Trevor	20	Seamstress	NAD	DI
Quick	23	Dispenser	NAD	Px
Crow	23	Secretary	PCO, early abortion	C
Menzies	34	Typist	NAD	Px
Holt	34	Housewife	Blocked tubes	C
Lamb	26	Typist	Endo, fibroids, PCO, asynch.	C
Diamond	28	Assembler	NAD	Px
Flower	23	Housewife	Blocked tube	P
Trafford	22	Beautician	Blocked tube, adhesions	(C)
David	28	Machinist	Blocked tube, adhesions, endo.	P
Neal	25	Cleaner	Oligomen., PCO	P
Mitchell	29	Teacher	Oligomen., endo.	DI
Newsome	29	Home help	Blocked tube	P

Key

Asynch.:	asynchronous menstrual cycle
PCO:	polycystic ovarian disease
C:	remained childless
P:	had a child after treatment
Px:	had a child without treatment

Endo.:	endometriosis
NAD:	no abnormality detected, within normal range
(C):	childless/separated
DI:	child via DI
Adop.:	adopted child

N.B. (a) terms defined in Glossary.

(b) basic investigations including HSG are not counted as treatment; laparoscopy is (see p. 82 below).

Table 4.3 Key characteristics: men

	Age	Occupation	Diagnosis	Outcome
Coleman	26	Production engineer	NAD	Px
Carver	34	Civil servant	Azoospermia	DI
Ivy	27	Accountant	NAD	P
Dorairaj	40	Accountant	NAD	C
Green	29	Care assistant	Oligospermia	C
Underwood	27	Shopkeeper	Azoospermia	C
Turner	29	Farm worker	Azoospermia	C
Truswell	26	Industrial engineer	Oligospermia	C
Young	32	Driver	Oligospermia	C
Thurston	22	Builder	NAD	Adop.
Grindrod	33	Foreman	Azoospermia	C
Monk	28	Computer programmer	NAD	P
Kitchen	33	Steel worker	NAD	C
Butler	33	Administrator	NAD	Px
Carter	26	Teacher	NAD	(C)
Urmston	39	Manager	Oligospermia	P
Keith	30	Electronics engineer	NAD (low normal)	P
Trevor	21	Machine operator	Oligospermia	DI
Quick	24	Welder	Oligospermia	Px
Crow	30	Manager	Oligospermia	C
Menzies	37	Welder	NAD	Px
Holt	31	Joiner	Oligospermia	C
Lamb	28	Computer programmer	NAD	C
Diamond	28	Printer	NAD	Px
Flower	30	Labourer	NAD	P
Trafford	29	Telephone engineer	NAD (low normal)	(C)
David	29	Fitter	NAD	P
Neal	25	Miner	NAD (low normal)	P
Mitchell	25	Chemist	Oligospermia	DI
Newsome	27	Bricklayer	NAD	P

Key: as in Table 4.2

Of the 30 couples, 22 (73 per cent) were both in their *first marriage*; four of the husbands had been married before, one of the wives, and both partners in three cases. In comparison with national figures, this suggested a slight bias to the more traditional patterns of marriage. As discussed in

Chapter 3, the dominant social norm is that children should be born within marriage. One illustration of this norm may be seen in the responses to the Family Practitioner Survey (FPS). Whilst 72 per cent of the doctors would refer a single woman for infertility investigation, only 57.5 per cent would refer a single man; strong evidence for the continued importance of this association. The decision in the case of the Holts, and the attitude of the family doctors, might suggest that this is one of the areas of selectivity in the referral of childless people to the Clinic.

The mean *duration of the couple's relationship* at the time of their first appointment at the Clinic was 58 months, median 52.5 (range 12 to 139). Amongst those couples where neither partner had previously been pregnant or fathered a child, the mean was 67.1 months. This suggested a very substantial delay in seeking medical help; the current median interval between marriage and first live birth was 28 months (OPCS 1986b).

Where *family building* was delayed, the couples declared a gap between starting the attempt to have a child and being referred to the Infertility Clinic of between 5 and 137 months – a mean of 26.7 and median of 20. As reported elsewhere, there is a large degree of unanimity in the literature that 12 months' uncontracepted, regular intercourse (in the absence of other significant factors such as advanced age or known pathology) is an appropriate period after which the couple might reasonably be said to display subfertility meriting specialist investigation. Almost half of the GPs responding to the FPS (46 per cent) claimed they would normally refer to a specialist when the couple had been trying for children for between 12 and 18 months; 12 months being the single most frequently reported period and the range being 2 to 24 months. The results in this study may represent that difficult gap between reported and actual behaviour, or there might be some effect in the strong bias of response within the FPS towards the younger GP. There is clearly a major discrepancy in this area. These couples, on average, were waiting twice this period before receiving specialist investigation of their fertility problem. This issue will be explored further in relation to the role of the GP.

Those who had previously been using the *contraceptive pill* were referred on average after 22.1 months compared with the whole group after 26.8 months. Evidence suggests there might be an interactive effect between age and oral contraception in impairing fertility, which might influence the earlier referral of these women.

Twenty-five (83 per cent) of the women, and the same percentage of the men, presented at the clinic with *primary infertility*, in the strict medical sense of not having already conceived (whether or not the child was born alive) or fathered a child. Of the five women with secondary infertility, four had previously had a termination of pregnancy, and one had a daughter.

This did not appear to be a greater matter of concern for the husbands involved than those cases in which the wife had not previously conceived. In the reverse case this seemed to increase the distress of the wife. (In two cases the abortion had been concealed from the husband, and I agreed not to raise the issue.) Of the five secondarily infertile men, four had children in a previous marriage. This emerged in the study as an important issue for the wife concerned; her infertility being perceived as 'failure' in contrast to the fertility of the ex-wife.

Only one couple belonged to an *ethnic minority*; the Dorairajes, who were originally from East Africa. This is statistically an accurate reflection of the population of the area, in which 3.2 per cent live in households headed by an individual born in the New Commonwealth or Pakistan (the most accurate measure of ethnicity available from the Census 1981), although it should be remembered that the ethnic minority population of the area is very much younger, and hence contains proportionately more at this family-building stage. However, on checking the notes of all Clinic patients at the time, it was found that 10 out of 123 new referrals were of Asian parentage. There were no Afro-Caribbeans. The lack of any Afro-Caribbean family doctors in Sheffield may be of significance. There was an African doctor working in the Clinic at the time, although this would not be widely known. Nearly all the Asian patients, from the name given, appeared to have been referred by an Asian doctor. Coombe (1976) has demonstrated the under-use of ante-natal services by ethnic minorities; although Townsend and Davidson (1982) and Black (1980) note only the lack of available evidence. Racism amongst referral agents, or anticipation of it amongst black people, could be factors, as could culturally distinct attitudes to fertility and the role of doctors. (For a discussion of these issues, the work in relation to mental health services by Aggrey Burke (Coombe and Little 1986) could be of equal relevance; see also Wilson 1981.) The ethnic minorities did appear to be under-represented in the Clinic.

They were not a *mobile group*, with 39 (65 per cent) of the respondents living within 20 miles of their birthplace. Fifteen couples moved house during the period of the study, but only two moved out of the same area.

The influence of certain *religions* on attitudes to fertility and the treatment of infertility was discussed in Chapter 3. It was striking that only three couples and one individual were active in a religion: 18 (60 per cent) of the men and 23 (77 per cent) of the women claimed nominal adherence to the Church of England; there were three Roman Catholics, only one claiming to be active in his religion. This picture suggests an under-representation of those committed to a religious organisation which might put obstacles in the path of investigation (e.g. Roman Catholics, Jews, fundamentalist black sects, Jehovah's Witnesses, Moslems).

From the details of *educational attainment*, it appeared that the men were substantially better qualified than the population as a whole. This was not the case for the women. The better educated women in the study group sought help for their infertility more quickly than those of lesser attainment.

There is a clear over-representation from the higher *social classes* (as measured by occupation of the husband) in the study group compared to the population at large. Connolly *et al.* (1987) record a similar, although slightly less atypical, class distribution. This class filter has been identified in the usage of all health services (Townsend and Davidson 1982). This effect might be strengthened in this case by the Clinic being a professorial unit in a teaching hospital. More working-class couples might be referred to district general hospital gynaecologists instead.

Only five (17 per cent) of the couples mentioned *financial problems*, although they all saw them as having no bearing on the decision to pursue a pregnancy. The majority had materially comfortable lifestyles.

Having adequate *housing* was cited by many of the couples as a key factor in the decision to have children. None of these couples was inadequately housed. Only seven (23 per cent) lived in council-owned accommodation, compared with 42.7 per cent of the population of South Yorkshire; a clear under-representation. This reinforces the picture of a predominantly higher social class and upwardly mobile group.

The *family size* of the study group was larger than might be expected if they simply reflected the wider population. Nine (15 per cent) of them were only children, and 18 (30 per cent) came from families with four or more children. These figures compare to the population estimate made in the General Household Survey 1966 (when most of the study group would have been with their parents) in which 42.6 per cent of families had an only child, and just 8.8 per cent had four or more children (OPCS 1968). The pressure exerted by families on these childless people will be discussed later. Clearly these couples felt siblings having children, and parents with no other expectations of grandchildren, as particularly strong sources of pressure.

In summary, the study group could not be said to be representative of the wider population. This picture tends to support the views of the Clinic staff that the patients are a socially selected group. This confirms the findings of Owens (1979, 1982) and Connolly *et al.* (1987) rather than those of Hull *et al.* (1985) and Rocker (1963).

Problems diagnosed

The individual detail may be found in Tables 4.2 and 4.3. The diagnoses are summarised here (Tables 4.4 and 4.5). Several of these diagnoses lack a clear line between what may be regarded as either 'normal' or 'pathological' – that is, they are matters of clinical judgement. Practice varies between clinics and practitioners on several dimensions, notably hormonal levels and sperm analyses. A judgement has been made in these cases on the basis of the medical notes and the advice of Professor Cooke. Azoospermia and amenorrhoea are examples of diagnoses which are unequivocal at a point in time but only sometimes permanent, untreatable and therefore final.

In comparing the outcome of investigation with the locus of the fertility problem, the results in Table 4.6 were found. The category 'child' includes those who conceived a child naturally and through DI.

Table 4.4 Problems diagnosed: women

	No.	*%*
Ovulatory/hormonal[1]	12	40
Structural[2]	8	27
Endometriosis/PCO	6	20
Psychosexual[3]	2	7
Nil[4]	11	37

Multiple problems gives totals in excess of 100 per cent

1. Irregular or absent ovulation, with or without regular menses, or a defect of hormone production, luteal phase, implantation or early development.
2. Blocked tubes, ovarian cysts, fibroids, adhesions.
3. Irregular intercourse, not timed to fertile period.
4. No abnormality detected, or abnormality judged not to be inhibiting conception.

Table 4.5 Problems diagnosed: men

	No.	*%*
Azoospermia[1]	4	13
Oligospermia[2]	10	33
Psychosexual[3]	2	7
Nil[4]	16	53

Multiple problems gives totals in excess of 100 per cent

1. No live sperm observed on at least two analyses, confirmed by testicular biopsy.
2. Impaired motility, count, progression or morphology.
3. Irregular intercourse, not timed to fertile period.
4. No abnormality detected/within normal range.

Table 4.6 Locus of fertility problem

	Child [1]		Childless		Total	
	No.	*%*	*No.*	*%*	*No.*	*%*
Male	3	10	3	10	6	20
Female	7	23	5	17	12	40
Both	2	7	6	20	8	27
Neither	4	13	0	0	4	13
Total	16	57	14	43	30	100

1. Child conceived naturally and/or with DI.

From these results, it is clear that the least successful outcome was in those cases in which both partners had a clearly identified problem. This is hardly surprising, but confirms the experience described in Rocker (1963), Philipp and Carruthers (1981), Wren (1985) and Winston (1986). The improved success with female problems only shows up as marginal in this sample, but also confirms the general experience (ibid.).

In the light of the discussion of the question of unexplained infertility, it is of interest that all of those for whom no problem was clarified conceived a child. Although they were classified here as having no problem, none of these situations was entirely unexplained. These cases are worth noting here;

Coleman: pregnant 5 months from intake, retroverted uterus and possible blockage of one tube, varicocele;

Butler: pregnant 7 months from intake, retroverted uterus and small fibroid, low motility but in normal range;

Menzies: pregnant 6 months from intake, possible endometrium problem;

Diamond: pregnant at intake, contraceptive pill for 6 years, HSG equivocal.

Progress of investigation

The period for which the members of the study group attended the Clinic, and the timing of interviews, is illustrated in Table 4.7 and Figure 4.1; from these it is clear that some of the respondents attended the Clinic for a substantial period of time; some were still attending, or on a waiting list after four years. The mean period was 18.6 months.

Table 4.7 Period attending Clinic

	No.	%
Less than 13 months	13	43
13–24 months	6	20
More than 24 months	11	37

There was no clear expectation as to how long the process might take: when they were asked at their first attendance, one-third of both men and women were unable to guess how long it might take; 14 (47 per cent) of the women and 13 (43 per cent) of the men expected to be attending the Clinic for periods of between 6 and 12 months; four men and four women (13 per cent) expected it to last in excess of 12 months. The estimates made ranged from a 'few weeks' to 'years'. It was noticeable that only five (17 per cent) of the couples agreed with each other within these bands in their estimate in answer to this question, suggesting a lack of communication between the couple as to their expectations. Clearly these estimates were well below what happened for a number of the couples.

It did not prove possible to obtain an accurate number of attendances at the Clinic; the respondents had frequently lost count, and the notes were not complete in every case – e.g. DI visits were not recorded, nor visits to other clinics in the same hospital for related help. It would be inaccurate to give the impression that the pattern of attendance was regular or similar for all; there were substantial variations according to the nature of the problem that was found and the treatment proposed. (It should be noted that in common with other aspects of the service at this Clinic, since the time of this research, the pattern of attendance and investigation has become much more rapid and standard. It is clear from reports in the pages of *Issue*, however, that the situation recorded here still obtains in many infertility services.)

Being a teaching hospital clinic, with a strong research commitment, meant that new investigations or treatments were frequently being introduced, some on an experimental basis. Patients had the choice of whether or not to be involved. On the whole, some of the qualities of this service seemed to be appreciated: the staff appeared to be at the forefront of developments; any new ideas were being made available; and the patients would not be missing anything that could be found elsewhere.

There seemed to be an acceptance of whatever was proposed by the Clinic, although the personal decision making will be discussed in detail later. The general attitude of the patients appeared to be that the Clinic

Figure 4.1 Progress of investigation

Name	Months
	10 20 30 40 50 60
	I.......+.......+.......+.......+.......+.......+
Coleman	P1 _ _ _ _ _ _ _ _ _ _ _ _ _ _ _ _ 2
Carver	1D _ _ _ _ _ _ P_ _ _ _ _ _ _ _ 2
Ivy	1 P _ _ _ _ _ _ _ _ _ _ _ _ _ _ _ _ 2
Dorairaj	1 X _ _ _ _ _ _ _ 2
Green	1 X _ _ _ _ _ _ _ _ _ _ _ 2
Underwood	1 X _ _ _ _ _ _ _ _ _ 2
Turner	1 D _ _ _ _ _ _ _ _ _ 2
Truswell	X1 _ _ _ _ _ _ _ _ _ _ _ _ _ _ _ _ 2
Young	X _ 1 _ _ _ _ _ _ _ _ _ 2
Thurston	1 > _ _ _ _ 2
Grindrod	1 D _ _ _ _ _ 2
Monk	1 X _ _ _ _ _ _ P_ 2
Kitchen	1 X _ _ _ _ _ _ 2
Butler	P 1 _ _ _ _ _ _ _ _ _ _ _ _ _ 2
Carter	X1 _ _ _ _ _ _ _ _ _ _ _ _ _ _ 2
Urmston	1 _ _ P _ _ _ _ _ _ _ 2
Keith	1 P _ _ _ _ _ _ _ _ 2
Trevor	D _ _ 1 _ _ _ _ _ _ P _ _ _ _ _ _ _ 2
Quick	P _ _ _ _ _ _ 1 _ _ _ _ _ _ 2
Crow	1 > _ 2
Menzies	P1 _ _ _ _ _ _ _ _ _ _ _ _ _ _ 2
Holt	1 2 X
Lamb	1 >2
Diamond	P _ _ _ 1 _ _ _ _ _ _ _ _ _ _ _ _ 2
Flower	1 P _ _ _ _ _ _ _ 2
Trafford	1 X _ _ _ _ _ _ _ 2
David	1 _ _ P_ _ _ _ _ 2
Neal	1 P _ _ _ _ _ 2
Mitchell	1 D P _ _ _ _ 2
Newsome	1 P _ _ 2
	I.......+.......+.......+.......+.......+.......+
	10 20 30 40 50 60

_____ months in treatment: mean 18.6 (range 0–48)

_ _ _ _ months in study: mean 45 (range 39–57)

Key

1/2	1st/2nd follow–up	P	Pregnant (last period)
>	continuing treatment or waiting list	D	DI waiting list
X	withdrew/refused further treatment	I	Intake

doctors were the experts in dealing with their problem, and they would know best what to provide. 'Whether to continue' was the patient's prerogative, and 'what treatment to provide' was the doctor's, would be a fair way of summarising the views of the patients in this matter. DI is the clear exception to this. The degree of this acceptance will be considered in relation to the study group's perceptions of their treatment. It is relevant to note at this point that there was little questioning of the advice received. One investigation, the testicular biopsy, was conducted without question in 9 of the 14 cases of sperm defects although it only led to treatment in one case, and on the whole it was used for the research material it obtained, not in the expectation that it was likely to lead to effective treatment. In one case, the Truswells, a traumatic biopsy was believed in the Clinic to have played a part in their withdrawing from treatment, although they did not report this themselves. This seemed a striking example of the passivity induced in the patients, not unique to this setting of medicine (Fitzpatrick 1984).

The question of private treatment only came up, interestingly, in connection with the much criticised waiting periods and frequent changes of doctor, not in anticipation of scientifically better treatment. Owens and Read (1979) report that 42 per cent of the childless people they surveyed went for private treatment at some stage, with 82 per cent initially seeking help from the NHS. In the context of this Clinic there was an infertility clinic run by many of the same staff, referred to as the University Clinic, which operated more consciously as a research facility. This clinic was similar to a private service in some respects. Only one of the couples in this study group was subsequently seen in the University Clinic.

Ovulation disorders requiring serial measurement of hormone levels and, latterly, ultrasound assessment of follicle development were examples of investigations allied to treatment which were very time consuming, and required very frequent attendance at the Clinic over limited periods. Many of the patients, whose problems were resolved or a final diagnosis reached fairly soon, would only attend on four to six occasions, however.

One striking finding was the difference in the experience of the women compared to their partners. Whilst there were those husbands who attended the Clinic almost as often as their wives, there were many others whose attendance was much less frequent. These differences will be discussed in more detail in Chapter 8. At this stage we might note that four (13 per cent) husbands never went at all, two (7 per cent) went to the Clinic but were never seen by medical staff, six (20 per cent) went on only one occasion; and the remaining 18 (60 per cent) went on at least one occasion. It is not suggested that the men simply had a lesser investment in the whole matter, although this was clearly the case for some. Rather it will be argued that a number of factors conspired to discourage the full participation of men in the process, which, overall, seemed to have a deleterious effect on the service and its impact on the couples concerned.

The decision to delay the final interview was clearly appropriate in giving a fairly comprehensive picture of their experience without it being too remote. As can be seen, there were only two couples who were actively pursuing more treatment when they were all interviewed for the last time. The mean period covered by the study for each couple was 45 months; the variation was accounted for by a range of circumstances including the pattern of events at the Clinic, personal crises and changes in their own lives as well as my own workload. The longest period was accounted for by the Greens, as can be seen from Figure 4.1. It took a long time to track them down after they moved house, and several failed visits before it was made clear that Mrs Green was unwilling to talk about their experiences. The circumstances are described in Chapter 8. The Truswells had moved away, forgetting to leave word. On one occasion I telephoned to confirm directions for the first follow-up interview that evening to be told by the breathless Mrs Quick that she had just gone into labour and was waiting for her husband to take her to the hospital. We agreed to postpone our interview! Overall it seemed that a balanced picture of the experiences of infertility patients was obtained.

Outcome and diagnosis

More than two-thirds of the couples were hopeful, when asked at initial interview, of being able to conceive a child through their attendance at the Clinic. It could be said that this is on the low side; having had oneself referred to a specialist clinic might be said to be an act of confidence that this is going to achieve the resolution of the problem.

Two-thirds of the women, although rather fewer men, felt positive enough to believe that most or nearly all of the patients would be able to have a child as a result of attending the Clinic. Only one of the men believed

Table 4.8 Outcomes

	No.	%
Pregnant after treatment	8	27
Pregnant after DI	3	10
Pregnant without treatment	5	17
Adopted	1	3
Childless	13	43
Total	30	100

that very few of the patients would achieve what they hoped for. The situation of the respondent couples at the conclusion of the study is summarised in Table 4.8.

The meaning of 'treatment' is not as precise as might be imagined in this field. For example, I have classified the HSG as an investigation, but it has been suggested that the action of the dye might make patent a slightly blocked fallopian tube. However, a laparoscopy has been identified as treatment: although the principal purpose of the laparoscopy is diagnostic, it was frequently used with a dye test, and the opportunity was taken, whilst the patient was under anaesthetic, to separate any minor adhesions or remove any small polyps noticed. The justification for regarding it as treatment was particularly in recognition of the importance, both thera-peutic and symbolic, attached to it by the patients. As it is the first of the procedures which requires hospitalisation and a general anaesthetic, it clearly assumed major importance in the minds of the patients. The 'heart searching' described by the Butlers most clearly demonstrated this. Of the men with sperm defects given testicular biopsies, only Mr Truswell was given treatment, hormone therapy, which proved ineffective and they remained childless.

Comparison with pregnancy rates at other clinics is unlikely to be of value as so much will depend on the nature of the population served; centres which attract the more complex cases on referral from generalist hospitals may not be able to reflect their greater success in higher overall rates of pregnancy. Stanway (1980) claims a rate in excess of 50 per cent as a guide, which would match the rate in this case. Rocker's (1963) rate of 34.5 per cent must in part be attributed to the dramatic development in medical knowledge in this field over the intervening period. Hull *et al.* (1985) claim a pregnancy rate of around 50 per cent and Philipp and Carruthers (1981) a rate of 65 per cent.

It could well be that other couples who remained childless at the end of the study period could still become pregnant or adopt a child. Two of these 13 couples were still being actively treated in the Clinic and the adoptive couple was on the waiting list for IVF. It is also possible that some of these couples might change their minds about further treatment, or be invited to consider re-entering treatment in the event of a development relevant to their needs. However, three of the husbands had been found to be azoospermic. Thus, with no chance of fertility and no prospect of dramatic treatments appearing for this condition, the only possible development for these couples would be for them to decide to accept DI, which they had thus far rejected. Their feelings about this approach will be considered later. After one unsuccessful course of DI one couple were on the waiting list for more, although uncertain about whether or not to proceed. One couple, the

Truswells, in which the man was oligospermic, decided to eliminate the uncertainty and remain childless by his having a vasectomy.

The possibility of future treatment remained for six of those where the woman had a difficulty. In two of the other cases the couple's marriage broke up, causing the cessation of treatment before a conclusion could be reached. In one case, the Holts' last remaining hope, IVF, was closed by the Clinic who decided that it was not possible to allocate them one of the scarce places in that expensive programme. Several reasons were advanced: Mrs Holt's age, 39; only one ovary available; Mr Holt also had a poor sperm count; the cost would be £300 per cycle; they were not married. (Professor Cooke's team argued the necessity of this last requirement at this early stage in the IVF programme, given the adverse publicity generated by such pregnancies in other programmes.)

In summary, the experience of the study group seems to have been representative of the Clinic population as a whole with regard to the outcome of their investigation and treatment.

5 Acknowledging childlessness

The first step in any form of medical treatment is the recognition that there is a problem, and, moreover, that it is a problem which can appropriately be taken to a doctor. This chapter concerns those couples who came to the Infertility Clinic and the ways in which they came to take this step. The Houghtons overstate the case in saying:

> It has to be remembered that infertility is primarily a *medical* problem.
> (Houghton and Houghton 1984: 21)

Even at the first stage, it is clear that infertility cannot be regarded as primarily medical, if one is to do justice to the perceptions childless couples have of their situation. In that the study group was recruited in the Infertility Clinic, the emphasis from this material will be the perspectives of those who decided to declare their childlessness a medical problem. The GPS has presented some data concerning those who did not make this choice.

CLINIC PATTERN

The couples whose experiences and views are discussed in this book attended the only local Infertility Clinic. Since the time of these interviews the operation of the Clinic has very substantially changed; although this is not a description of the Clinic as it now operates, the National Association for the Childless (*Issue* No. 21, 1991) found that 4:5 of the calls to their helpline were complaining of poor standards in the infertility clinics consulted by their members.

On each Tuesday afternoon on which the Clinic was held, in the Antenatal Clinic, three or four new patients would be offered appointments at 15-minute intervals from two o'clock onwards, the appointments having been sent out on standard gynaecology out-patients cards marked 'Hospital for Women', and addressed to the woman alone. After booking in with the reception staff, the woman was asked to provide a urine specimen, then undress completely, changing into an operation gown. She would then be expected to remain in a small cubicle, awaiting the call to see the doctor. If the male partner was present, he would sit on his own in the general waiting area. In view of the 15-minute interval between appointments, and the fact that the doctor's examination and recording of the history would take from 30 to 45 minutes in most cases, those with the later appointments could wait for two hours before being seen. On occasion, when there were difficulties with medical cover, patients had waited four hours, but this was exceptional.

During this waiting period I would introduce myself to those patients who appeared to meet the research criteria, according to the information contained in the medical notes or GP's referral letter. The woman would be told that a survey was being conducted with the help of patients attending the Clinic, and agreement to an interview sought. If the patient raised no objection at this stage, a brief note was given which explained in more detail the purposes of the research, and the patient was asked to look out for me after the conclusion of the interview with the doctor, before leaving to make an appointment with the radiography department (for an HSG, hysterosalpingogram – see Appendix III), which was the final element of the routine.

The interview with the doctor would include physical examination, taking a detailed history, and finally a blood sample. If the partner was present, usually he would then be interviewed, and a history taken, and physical examination performed. This routine was much less predictable than that for the woman. Although it was the stated intention of the Clinic to investigate the man as fully as the woman from the start, one registrar, an Asian woman doctor, on no occasion during my attendance at the Clinic asked to see the man. If the woman patient asked for him to be seen, she would take a history but not undertake physical examination. Other registrars also appeared to take the view that a physical examination would only be undertaken in the event of the semen analysis proving to be deficient in some respect. This attitude seemed to reinforce the dominant ideology referred to elsewhere, which stresses the primacy of the woman's responsibility for infertility investigation, despite the fact that the difficulty is as likely to lie with the male as with the female partner (Winston 1990).

After dressing, the woman would in most cases be required to receive instruction from a nurse on the method of taking her basal body temperature for completion of the temperature charts, one of the basic investigations undertaken. She would then have to see reception staff to make the follow-up appointment suggested by the doctor, before leaving the Clinic for the radiography department. I would intercept the patient(s) once again for initial interview before she or they left the Clinic.

READINESS TO PARENT

As was noted in Chapter 3, the evidence available suggests that parenting is so much perceived as a 'normal' part of marriage – or in certain cultural settings, courtship – that for many couples the question 'why' or 'if' to have children is hardly asked.

It would have been insensitive to ask the couples in this study 'why'; they were, however, asked for the reasons they decided to try for children at that particular time. The answers were the prosaic ones noted by Busfield and Paddon (1977) (see Table 5.1):

Table 5.1 Readiness for parenthood

	No.	*%*
Sound financial position	9	30
Home ready	6	20
Relationship settled	3	10
Wanted children a.s.a.p.	18	60

Multiple replies gives totals in excess of 100 per cent.

The almost two-thirds who 'simply' wanted children clearly saw the contraction of marriage as the decision to become parents, and that family = children.

> No particular reason, we wanted to be a family.   (Mrs Truswell)

The only reason for delay was the need to:

> Get straightened round, ready for children.   (Mr Kitchen)

Amongst the other reasons offered were: the age of the wife in two cases of substantial delay; doctors suggesting, for medical reasons, that delay was inadvisable; the hoped for time of birth matched career needs for two of the professional women in the study; the 'example' of friends and relatives. There was little to suggest a carefully planned sequence of events.

They appeared to share socially typical intentions of family size: 23 women (77 per cent) and 24 men (80 per cent) envisaged one or two children at the time of marriage. Only one woman and two men had not intended to have any children. There was a large measure of agreement between spouses as to the number of children intended at this time (77 per cent). At this stage there was little revising of the number of children the couples expected; only two of the women were conscious of lowered expectations, whilst three of the men and one woman felt they now wanted more children than they had expected at the time of marriage. The anxiety of these couples to have children did not express itself in terms of unusually large family size. In this respect they seemed fairly typical of other couples (Cartwright 1976, Dunnell 1979).

Asked when they first became concerned, 14 (47 per cent) said within 12 months of first trying to conceive. Six (20 per cent) gave a period of 13–18 months. The three who gave periods in excess of this gave 24, 48 and 54 months. Five couples (17 per cent) noted that they had suspected the existence of a problem from the beginning because of factors in their medical history. The Keiths were the only couple to say that they did not feel concerned at any time, but had sought referral simply in order to explain the failure to conceive.

Few specific reasons were identified as causing the couple to feel concerned at a particular time. Twelve (40 per cent) said it was simply a matter of time passing. Eleven (37 per cent) felt the age of the wife was a matter of some concern.

> If the wife was 22, we wouldn't be here now.   (Mr Carver)

Other prompts were the discussions the couple had (two), the prompting of friends in three cases, the husband's mother in two cases and the Family Planning Clinic in one case.

> Pressure from the in-laws is getting quite intense; my brother and his wife have had two in the time we've been trying.   (Mr Mitchell)

> People did joke about it; 'Don't you want a family?' We didn't admit the problems. It all upset me.   (Mrs David)

Six (20 per cent) of the respondent couples mentioned growing anxiety as an important factor; a matter to which I shall return.

INITIAL ADVICE

Where did the childless couples first turn for advice, or at least, for an opportunity to share the information that they were having difficulty in conceiving the child they wanted? The lapse of time that occurred has already been described. This is the point at which the 'accommodation' described by Zola (1973) is breaking down, and the couple are preparing to make the admission that they are involuntarily childless to themselves and to selected other people, crucially their doctors.

Not surprisingly, all of the wives said that they normally first discuss things 'on their minds' with their husband, although four mentioned their mothers and four friends or a sister as taking this role. Twenty-seven (90 per cent) of the men also said they first talked to their wives, only three also mentioned friends, and two family. Three of the men made a point of saying they kept things to themselves as much as possible. Four (13 per cent) of the women but 14 (47 per cent) of the men had told no one else about the apppointment at the Infertility Clinic. The general picture was one of greater reluctance amongst the men to discuss the fertility problems outside the marriage, or the immediate family. Such reluctance would obviously mirror stereotypes of 'male' behaviour in our society (Eichenbaum and Orbach 1983). However, it has to be said that no more men than women (seven, 23 per cent) admitted to being unable to discuss their difficulties in having children easily, or feeling that discussing the situation made it easier to cope with (five, 17 per cent).

In only three instances did either partner mention having first shared their concern with someone other than the partner. In two cases this was the GP, and in one case, Mrs Holt, the adult daughter. Five (17 per cent) of the men and six (20 per cent) of the women next confided in their GP. Parents or parents-in-law were confided in by eight (27 per cent) of the men and seven (23 per cent) of the women at the second stage. The significant differences between the partners emerged in relation, firstly, to the use of friends in the role of confidant, four (13 per cent) men but eight (27 per cent) women; and, secondly, to those who had confided in no one other than the partner, ten (33 per cent) men and six (20 per cent) women. It was surprising perhaps that only five (8 per cent) of the respondents, men and women, said that the first person they confided in other than the spouse was the wife's mother. This is at variance with the central role ascribed to her by Oakley (1979) and Cartwright (1976). It should be noted that in most cases this question was asked of the couple together: this may have inhibited replies which might not have been welcomed by the spouse, although I have no evidence of this effect. There was evidence in the opposite direction: the Truswells showed considerable surprise, and some annoyance, when each stated that they had discussed their childlessness with their own friends – something they had not admitted before the interview. Mrs Truswell had also been to the GP before discussing it with her husband.

He played hell with me for going to see the doctor without telling him.

Almost without exception these contacts were felt to be helpful, not for the advice they offered, but for the simple concern and understanding received. Naturally they will only have confided in those they expected would be sympathetic; the attitudes of others were not always so empathic, as will be discussed later. The simple helpfulness of talking was often mentioned, in this context, as well as in relation to the interviews for the research. Only in one instance did I record in my comments on the first interview that, whilst the couple verbally maintained that it had been helpful to confide in the people they mentioned and also to talk to me, they gave every indication in other replies that they had talked to each other very little. This couple, the Traffords, separated three years later.

When asked to rate the attitudes of others to their difficulties, the women seemed to feel slightly more positive than the men. However, when asked which parts of their social network (family, friends, work colleagues) knew of their fertility problems, it was apparent that the men confided in fewer people than the women in the study.

The couples seemed to have received very little relevant advice from their confidants. Only ten (33 per cent) reported any advice; this ranged from the magical or exotic:

More sex, Guinness and goat skin rugs!   (Mrs Truswell)

through urging to relax, and 'stop trying too hard', to the more practical advice about the fertile period offered by only two mothers who were trained nurses. The only other advice was to go to the doctor. The clear impression was of a reluctance to discuss their infertility problem, other than with the closest friends and relatives; and even these contacts seemed to help almost entirely by their concern, rather than by offering practical advice.

Judging from the responses to asking what they had tried that might improve their chances of conception, it seemed that some of these couples could have benefited from some practical advice. Sixteen (53 per cent) had changed nothing specifically. Others had tried a variety of things. The most common tactic was to time intercourse to the most fertile period. This was tried by six (20 per cent) couples, but two of these wives noted that this only served to 'work me up'. One of the three (10 per cent) who reported trying to relax and not think about conception too much commented sourly:

It's easier said than done!

In all, 11 ideas were mentioned a total of 27 times, most of which were sensible: taking wife's temperature, fertile period, regular sexual intercourse, reading expert advice, man wearing loose underwear, woman resting after intercourse. The only slightly unusual ideas were those to vary the position, place and time of day for intercourse mentioned by two couples. One tried herbal remedies and another Vitamin E. There was little evidence that most couples were being given, or that they were heeding, sensible, practical advice on maximising chances of conception. The reluctance to engage in discussions that would have made this possible clearly lay with the couples themselves as much as with those to whom they turned. It established a pattern of isolation which became very important for a significant proportion of these couples.

ENCOUNTERING THE GP

Not surprisingly, the first visit to the GP at which the couple's difficulty in conceiving was discussed, was a significant occasion for the respondents.

In 18 (60 per cent) cases the woman went on her own to see the GP in the first instance; in all others they went together, although two of the husbands simply sat in the waiting room whilst the wife saw the GP. One wife reported that their GP's receptionist refused to make an appointment for them to see the GP together, confirming one of the bleaker findings of Arber and Sawyer's study of doctors' receptionists (1985) that they too frequently make independent decisions about clinical matters. In no case did the husband go alone, notwithstanding the amount of distress the wife was said to be in, or those cases where there was known to be a likely problem on the man's side from his history. Perhaps it might be expected in the four cases of the man having already fathered a child in a previous relationship that the woman should initially go to the GP on her own. There were five couples in which the woman had herself previously conceived, suggesting some likelihood (although no certainty) of the problem being on the man's side, in four of these it was still the woman who went on her own to see the GP; their husbands never went to the GP for this reason.

In 13 (43 per cent) cases there was a delay of at least six months between the time when the couple reported becoming concerned and their seeing the GP. Various reasons were advanced to explain this further delay. Six (20 per cent) could offer no particular reason beyond a general reluctance. The attitude of the husband was also important here, in that two wives went without their husbands knowing in the first instance; in the case already quoted this caused some ill feeling, but not apparently in the other. Two mentioned pressures from the family as significant in making them take this step. Three cited other illness as creating the opportunity to raise the matter of failing to conceive. In all, 13 (43 per cent) went with another medical complaint on the first occasion. Both these findings suggest some reluctance to define fertility problems as sufficient cause to 'bother' their doctors.

The majority of the couples (or the wives who went on their own) felt positively about the reception given them by their family doctors. Twenty-four (80 per cent) made positive comments about the encounter. A number used the description 'sympathetic'.

> He was very sympathetic; took me more seriously than I expected, just referred me to the Clinic without much discussion.   (Mrs Truswell)

> Helpful, super; he's an excellent GP; he was keen to get on in view of
> my age.   (Mrs Butler)

Six (20 per cent) couples felt unhappy about their treatment by the GP. The
criticism was largely of a perceived lack of concern or interest.

> Not helpful at all. He just said 'keep on trying'; wanted to finish just as
> soon as possible. We wanted time; he didn't refer us on, asked nothing
> at all. He knew nothing about us at all. Ended up with him saying 'We'll
> see your wife at the ante-natal clinic soon'.   (Mr Dorairaj)

In comparison with the findings of Cartwright and Anderson (1981), this
could be said to be a slightly low level of satisfaction. Asking the views of
their sample patients on the care they received from their GP found 49 per
cent very satisfied and 42 per cent satisfied, with just 9 per cent having
mixed feelings or being dissatisfied.

Dissatisfaction did not directly correlate with the activity level of the
GP; five of the six who were not satisfied were examined, given advice or
a test, in addition to being referred on to the Infertility Clinic.

In the great majority of cases, 27 (90 per cent), the GP was said to have
been first to suggest referral to a specialist. In all but two of those cases, the
GP decided to whom they would be referred. The GP's role was clearly
very significant in this respect. The amount of contact with the GP prior to
referral to the Clinic may be seen from Table 5.2. As with other aspects of
the process, it will be noticed that the involvement of the men was substantially less than that of the women.

Two-thirds of the men saw the GP once or not at all, whilst almost the
same proportion of the women went twice or more often. The period over
which these consultations took place ranged from two weeks to 15 months.
In two cases there was a very much longer period caused by a 'lost'
appointment (19 months) and by not following up the consultation with the
GP, but leaving matters until the Family Planning Clinic made the referral
(four years). The mean period was five months for those cases, excluding
the extreme ones mentioned, in which referral was not made on the first
consultation.

The delay caused by waiting lists for the Infertility Clinic varied over the
period of the research due to factors including demand, staff shortages and
industrial action (Table 5.3). For these couples the delay between trying for
children and attending the Infertility Clinic comprised three 'delays' which
varied in relative length: waiting to consult the GP; seeing the GP; waiting
for the Clinic appointment. There was no standard ratio between these
periods, as has been indicated. It was, however, clear that most of the
couples felt that a lot of waiting was involved at this stage. Even where the

Table 5.2 Consultations with GP

No. of Consultations	Men		Women	
	No.	%	No.	%
Nil	13	43	0	0
1	7	23	13	43
2	5	17	12	40
3	4	13	4	13
4	1	3	1	3

Table 5.3 Delay to appointment

	No.	%
<3 months	9	30
3+4 months	13	43
5+6 months	8	27

GP had been involved in preliminary investigations, the perceptions of the patients of this period might best be described as one of 'marking time' before the 'real' investigation began.

LAY ADVICE

Given the perception of this waiting period as one of considerable stress and frustration, one might have expected the couples to make considerable use of friends and relatives in the role of confidants. Some of the support and advice offered to those who sought help before going to see their GP has already been described. Only 13 (43 per cent) of the men admitted looking to anyone other than the wife or GP for help and advice during this time. Rather more of the women took this course, 20 (67 per cent). This reflects the often remarked greater proclivity amongst women to discuss personal matters (e.g. Cartwright 1976, Cartwright and Anderson 1981, Scambler and Scambler 1984). A typical comment from one of the 17 men who kept it to themselves was:

> I'm not bothered [= *do not like*] talking to other people about it; I know others who've kept it quiet.   (Mr Diamond)

Several couples made the same point to me, expressed in the words of one of the husbands thus:

No one knows as much as we've told you.

Even amongst those who had discussed things with someone, several made a point of saying that the discussions had been very brief or entirely at the initiative of the other party.

The women offered a rather different picture. Not only had more of them confided in this way, but it seemed that the circle of confidantes was wider. Owens (1979) noted the important role of 'the girls at work' to the women he interviewed; this seemed important to a number of these wives also. No attempt was made to quantify the number of people involved in this confiding circle, but it appeared to be the case that quite a number of people were involved for some of the women respondents, but none of the men.

The advice given was similar to that already discussed, both in nature and scope. Rather than feeling able to use some of the advice, one woman noted:

It upsets me that most of the advice is given by people who've got children. (Mrs Newsome)

In summary, it would be fair to say that these couples, with the exception of those two who had a trained nurse in the family, saw discussions with family and friends as sources of support and understanding, used with some reticence, rather than as sources of relevant and helpful, practical advice.

GP REFERRAL

We may now look at the experience of consulting a GP about infertility, and the steps which this led to in the experience of the study group, as well as the practice reported by GPs in the FPS.

Table 5.4 records, for each of the respondents, who the doctor referred (i.e. woman alone or her husband also), the summarised details given in the referral letter, who actually attended the Clinic for the first appointment, and details of any investigations or treatment which the doctor said, or implied had been undertaken already. Explanation of the terms may be found in the Glossary.

Only in four (13 per cent) cases was the referral of the couple, rather than just the woman, in contradiction to the assertions of both texts and popular works on infertility, as well as to the stated intentions of this Clinic. This seemed particularly anomalous where the only information contained in the referral letter was that the husband was azoospermic. It was not, however, surprising that not all the husbands attended on the first appointment when it is recalled that the Infertility Clinic operated under the aegis of a gynae-cologist and obstetrician, based in a women's hospital. The appointment card was sent in the name of the woman only and the location of the Clinic was the ante-natal clinic. (All of these practices have changed at this Clinic since the time of this study, although certainly not at others.)

When the couple was jointly referred, in each case the man attended the Clinic as well. In all, the men accompanied their wives in 17 (57 per cent) cases. The feelings of husbands regarding their involvement in the process will be considered later.

When the GPs were asked about their practice, 69.5 per cent said that they referred the couple; a striking difference to the situation encountered at the Clinic where only four (13 per cent) were thus referred. All of the eight GPs in practices which they themselves described as predominantly middle class or professional would only refer patients as a couple. This did not mirror the consultation with the GP reported by the Clinic patients entirely. Twelve (40 per cent) of the couples went to the GP together to discuss their failure to conceive. In all the other cases the wife went alone on the first occasion. In 11 (37 per cent) cases the husband was never seen by the GP, although all but three had the same doctor. A clear impression is given that whatever specialists say about the intra-marital nature of infertility, the initiative is often taken by the woman, and the practice of GPs serves to support this situation.

To which specialist did GPs refer? A third of the GPs said that they referred infertility patients to this Clinic – half, if the non-specific answers just naming the hospital are included. A third simply refer to a gynaecologist. In practice this could mean the same thing, of course. These figures seemed surprisingly low for a city in which the only infertility clinic in the region was located. A similar percentage of men, a third, would be referred to this Clinic according to the GPs, although a further third would be referred to a urologist despite the lack of interest in infertility matters amongst the local urologists, who themselves would refer on to the Infertility Clinic.

There was evidence that more recently qualified doctors were twice as likely to refer both male and female patients direct to the Infertility Clinic than their longer serving colleagues; about 40 per cent in each case.

Lack of detail was perhaps the most striking thing about the referrals of these couples to the Infertility Clinic. All but one were made by the family doctor. In some cases the information amounted to no more than that the woman concerned was unable to conceive. The most frequent item of information offered, not surprisingly, was whether or not the patient had previously conceived. Twenty-six (87 per cent) gave this information, although in two of the five cases in which the man had previously fathered a child this information was not given. In one case the GP either did not

Table 5.4 Referral details

Name	Who was referred?	Details given	Who attended?	Investigated/ treated?
Coleman	W	1°, ovulation seems OK 16 mths since ceasing OC	B	
Carver	B	1°, 2 yrs. H. azoospermic	B	SA
Ivy	W	1°, 1 yr anovulatory, dysmenorrhoea OC 1 yr, long cycle	B	BBT
Dorairaj	B	1°, 20 mths, sperm count OK, normal menses, pelvis NAD	B	SA, Phys W
Green	B	low sperm count	B	SA
Underwood	W	subfertile 'got upset, please reassure'	W	
Turner	W	Azoospermic	B	SA
Truswell	W	2, 1 yr, previous contraception 6 yrs TOP	B	
Young	B	1°, previous TOP	B	
Thurston	W	1°, 1 yr, irregular periods	W	
Grindrod	W	1°, 11 yrs, infrequent sex, marital problems (ref. by FPC)	W	
Monk	W	1°, 2½ yrs, OC 7 yrs	B	
Kitchen	W	1°, 5 yrs	W	
Butler	W	1°, 1 yr	W	
Carter	W	1°, 6 mths, some problems with cont.	W	
Urmston	W	1°, 3 yrs, irregular menses, H child prev. marriage	B	BBT
Keith	W	1°, H. exposed to radiation at work	W	
Trevor	W	1°, 8 mths, amenorrhoea low sperm count	B	SA
Quick	W	1°, 18 mths, ovarian cyst removed as child, irregular menses	B	
Crow	W	1°, c.1 yr, prev. menstrual problems	B	
Menzies	W	1°, 2 yrs menarche 12, cycle 4/25–34 no dysmenorrhoea, SA normal	W	SA
Holt	W	Both have child prev. marriages, menstruation OK, no probs known	W	
Lamb	W	1°, 5 yrs.	W	
Diamond	W	1°, 18 mths off OC, short periods, married 7 yrs	B	
Trafford	W	1°, 18 mths off OC TOP 1974 H child prev. marriage	W	
Flower	W	1°, 3½ yrs, 2nd marriage 6 mths 'otherwise healthy'	W	
David	W	4½ yrs trying since marriage ovarian cyst removed 'concerned'	W	
Neal	W	1°, irregular periods	B	
Mitchell	W	1°, 18 mths, prev 2 yrs. OC, 'fit' Sex 2/3 p.w.	B	
Newsome	W	1°, 18 mths, regular menses/sex, OC prev. no rel. history, on tranx	B	SA, BBT

Key

W	Wife;	H	Husband	OC	Oral contraceptive
B	Both			SA	Semen analysis
1°	Primary infertility			BBT	Basal body temperature chart
2°	Secondary infertility			FPC	Family Planning Clinic
NAD	No abnormality detected			PhysW	Physical exam of woman

know, or failed to pass on, that the woman had previously undergone a termination. In two cases the meaning of primary infertility appeared to be idiosyncratic, being used to refer to two women who had previously conceived.

The next most common item of information offered was the period over which there had been a failure to conceive, 22 (73 per cent) of the letters; although it should be said that there was substantial disagreement between the figure given by the GP and that given to me by the respondents. There are substantially fewer referrals giving other important information: menstrual history/details of ovulation, 12 (40 per cent); contraceptive history, 9 (30 per cent); details of sperm quality, 6 (20 per cent); sexual history, 3 (10 per cent); and other relevant medical history, 10 (33 per cent).

Perhaps the most surprising omission is discussion of sex. For all the popular talk of permissiveness in society in relation to sexual matters, there was nothing in this study to support the view that these matters are in fact freely discussed, although no one would deny their importance. In reviewing the medical notes, the same reluctance was apparent. Whilst it is part of the agreed protocol for the first appointment, there were many cases in which information about the patients' sexual practices was not recorded. Only one-third of the notes contained this information. Given the experience of one couple, this reluctance appeared seriously to weaken the service of the Clinic. The Grindrods were referred as having substantial problems in relation to their sexual relationship by the Family Planning Clinic, but this seemed to rate very little attention. Indeed, the process of investigation appeared to continue in exactly the same way as for other couples. The problem was never considered separately; at the final interview, the couple were on the waiting list for DI.

The only couple to be referred for marital and sexual counselling, the Carters, presented their sexual difficulty simply as evidence of the severe difficulties in their relationship, rather than a separate, pre-existing matter. The different social status of the two couples might not be irrelevant here; the Carters being both in professional occupations, the Grindrods being manual workers, with the expected differences in levels of education and articulateness. The literature evaluating the work of counselling services universally draws attention to the greater likelihood of Young, Attractive, Verbal, Intelligent, Treatable people (YAVITs) being offered the 'talking treatments' than Humble, Old, Unattractive, Non-verbal, Depressed people (HOUNDs) (Smale 1977).

It should be noted that the case for the GP giving a very detailed referral is not uncontroversial. Whatever the GP said, or whichever results of investigations were given, the Clinic would often proceed with the usual pattern of investigation. The Clinic understandably wanted to use its own expertise and known laboratory facilities rather than take the opinion of others. One imagines that this would be a common view for medical specialists to take, on the argument that to do otherwise would undermine their very *raison d'être*. There were, for example, serious deficiencies in the way in which semen samples were evaluated in the local NHS laboratories at the time. No doubt this view would also be held by many of the GPs referring, inclining them to investigate little before onward referral. As will be discussed later, there was little expectation amongst the patients that the GP would do very much before passing them on to specialist help, indeed a common benchmark of the GP's concern was the speed with which such a referral was made. This does go against current trends which emphasise a major role for the primary care services.

The doctors replying to the FPS (Table 5.5) claimed to seek rather more information than typically was passed to the Clinic in the cases studied: 80.3 per cent said that they asked for three or more items of information from patients consulting with an infertility problem. Even more striking was the weight placed on various factors.

Unfortunately, limitations of space on the questionnaire meant that the questions could not be made as precise as desirable. In this case it is difficult to categorise answers accurately: 'gynaecological history' could well have meant to the answering doctor, 'previous conceptions' included. 'Past medical/surgical history' could include virtually everything else. It is nonetheless remarkable that much greater importance was attached to issues of sex than was accorded by the referring GPs or, it must be said, the Clinic. The main focus of concern in relation to sex was the frequency of intercourse. Given the frequent complaint of infertility specialists

Table 5.5 Information asked on infertility referral (FPS)

	No.	%
Details of intercourse/sexual history	84	63.2
Past medical/surgical history	75	56.4
Period of unprotected intercourse/'trying'	71	53.3
Menstrual history	35	26.3
Fertility history/previous conceptions	32	24.0
Current general health	26	19.5
Contraceptive history	26	19.5
Gynaecological history	25	18.8
Length of marriage/relationship	21	15.8

Multiple replies give totals in excess of 100 per cent.

Table 5.6 Investigation practice (FPS)

	No.	*%*
Physical examination	87	65.4
Semen analysis	50	37.6
Basal body temperature chart	50	37.6
Nil	31	23.3

Multiple replies gives totals in excess of 100 per cent.

concerning the extent of simple ignorance of the facts of reproduction (discussed in relation to the causes of infertility), it is still interesting that only ten GPs (7.5 per cent) mention the timing of sexual intercourse specifically. There was statistical significance in the association between the number of items of information a GP would seek and his or her being younger (χ^2=22.05, P=0.001) and having fewer years in general practice (χ^2=21.87, P=0.034). As in other responses, the evidence was that women GPs were no more active than men in their practice in these situations.

A similar picture emerged in relation to preliminary investigations undertaken. As can be seen from Table 5.4, the study group appeared, from the referral letters analysed, to have been little investigated before being referred to the Infertility Clinic. In seven cases (23 per cent) a semen analysis was conducted; in three (10 per cent), temperature charts were begun; in only one case was a physical examination mentioned. A rather different picture emerged in the interviews at which nine (30 per cent) said that a semen analysis had been done; in eight (27 per cent), BBT charts had been started; and in eight cases (27 per cent) there had been a physical examination of the wife. Only ten (33 per cent) said that nothing had been done other than the referral. In the FPS doctors claimed substantial rates of initial investigation, just over half saying they would undertake two or more investigations prior, or in addition, to referral. Again this was found to be positively associated with fewer years in practice (χ^2=13.31, P=0.001) and also younger age (τ_s=−0.2235, P=0.01). The most frequent investigations mentioned are itemised in Table 5.6.

Fifteen GPs (11.3 per cent) claimed to assess endocrine/hormonal function, a difficult and expensive investigation. The rigour of preliminary investigation suggested by these answers was not represented in the experience of the Clinic. A total of 123 referrals were checked, most of those received at this time. The nature of these referrals was apparently no different from the ones analysed; indeed, in the case of those referred for second opinions, the paucity of information was the more striking for the extent of the previous investigation undertaken but only briefly recorded. (It is likely that GPs in these cases would expect the Clinic to obtain previous hospital records, although frequently the detail of where the patient was previously investigated was missing.) The exceptions to this picture of thin referrals were those referred by other hospital consultants, usually gynaecologists, which were excluded from the study group.

The issue of the treatment the GP might offer is also controversial. As already mentioned, it would be quite wrong to give the impression that the conscientious GP *should* undertake certain treatments before referring on to a specialist. In the field of infertility the investigations require careful assessment before any course of treatment is undertaken, and many of the GPs replying felt that it would be premature for them to start any treatment before the specialised assessment. In the Clinic group none had been offered any treatment prior to referral, even where a problem was known. Amongst the GPs, 38 (29.7 per cent) said they would offer no treatment, or 85 (66.4 per cent) including those who would only refer the patient to a specialist. An equal proportion of male and female doctors adopted this course. 22 (17.2 per cent) suggested various forms of advice and counselling as the treatment they would offer. (This is one of the ambiguities in this question; there could well have been GPs who considered this contribution as too obvious to require stating, or worth regarding as 'treatment'.) Seven (23 per cent) of the study group felt they received this service, however. In Owens and Read's study (1979) 51 per cent claimed to have received some sort of practical advice from their GPs. The FPS GPs made a range of interesting comments on this question, including:

There is not any I can do, is there?

Stop the valium. [*N.B.* The Newsome's GP did the reverse.]

I would call in local authority help by advising such couples to get appropriate forms with a view to adoption of infants unwanted by their natural mother.

A few, more 'scientific', suggestions were also made. The comments about adoption, although made by only three out of 133 GPs, are of some concern in appearing to show ignorance of the adoption situation discussed in Chapter 1.

Overall, it could be said that there was substantial support amongst the GPs for seeing the matter of infertility investigation as one for the specialists. This could be said to lend support to the concern raised in the experience of the Clinic couples that GPs are not using to the full their knowledge of the process of conception which might serve to alleviate anxiety, avoid unnecessary referral, and perhaps ensure that those who did not pursue specialist help nonetheless received basic assistance.

PREPARATION FOR INVESTIGATION

The practical steps taken by the GP and the couple themselves to prepare for the specialist investigation at the Infertility Clinic have been discussed. Another measure of this is the knowledge held by the couple of the process that will be involved, and the difficulties that are to be addressed. It should be repeated that many of these interviews were conducted at a time of great stress for the couple; that is, the first appointment at the Infertility Clinic. This might well have artificially depressed their ability to answer this question; although there was little evidence that this could wholly explain the gaps in their understanding.

The couples were asked to state any factors they were aware of that could cause infertility. A variety of things were mentioned: 48 responses were given concerning male infertility, covering 11 items – a mean response of 1.6 items. A low sperm count was mentioned 17 times (57 per cent). In addition, ten other factors were mentioned at least once, all of which could be said to be explanations of poor sperm quality: hormones (2); mumps (12); veins, i.e. varicocoeles (2); drug/alcohol abuse (2); tight underwear (4); infections/disease (4); psychological problems (1); impotence (1); age (1); and 'physical' problems (1). Although the precise role of some of these factors is controversial, as discussed in Chapter 2, this suggested a level of information, and no irrational or fanciful explanations. It might be suggested that this question was differently understood; where the response was simply 'low sperm count', the couple was pressed to be more precise. Four couples were not able to be more specific. Taken with the five couples who were unable despite prompting to give any explanation for male infertility, this gave nine (30 per cent) without any prior grounding in the simple facts of their situation.

The knowledge of female factors in infertility was possibly a little better; but the larger number of factors mentioned should be put alongside the larger number of known factors from which to choose. Thirteen factors were mentioned a total of 60 times; a mean rate of response of 2 per couple. In order of the frequency with which they were mentioned, these factors were: tube problems (22), ovulation failure (15), disease/infections (4), physical abnormality (3), psychological problems (3), genetic problems (3), hormones (2), sex/incompatibility (2), previous abortion (2), abdominal operations (1), anaemia (1), 'chemicals' (1), pills (1). As with male factors, those mentioned were realistic, although the responses 'pills' and 'chemicals' were both entirely unspecific. Rather fewer couples said they knew of none (two, or 7 per cent), but nine could only mention one item, and just two were able to mention five items. Neither of the two women to mention the possible influence of abortion had themselves undergone the procedure.

They were also asked what they expected would be involved in terms of investigations or tests and treatments in their attendance at the Clinic. A rather more encouraging picture appeared here.

In relation to the male component, quite correctly 24 (80 per cent) expected to undergo semen analysis. There were 11 other responses: blood test (7), drugs (2), physical examination (1) and 'vein check' (1). The lack of expectation of active treatment was a fair anticipation of their actual experience; see Appendix III. Only one couple mentioned the post-coital test, which, despite the prominence given to it at other clinics, was little used here. This is discussed in Appendix III. Only two couples mentioned artificial insemination, which subsequently assumed considerable prominence in some cases; neither of these concerned the two men referred by the GP as being azoospermic. In four cases the couple could think of no test or treatment that would be involved.

Again, their responses in relation to the woman accurately reflected the greater variety of investigations and treatments available, in which the woman would be expected to participate. Eleven responses were given, although in surprising numbers. The most frequently mentioned item, 28 couples (93 per cent), was an X-ray; this includes the four who mentioned the hysterosalpingogram by name or implication. Given the anxiety of this first encounter with the Clinic, it could simply be that this description of the first investigation routinely performed – 'an X-ray of your tubes', used by Clinic staff as shorthand for the HSG – was simply the most easily recognised, and therefore recalled, piece of medical information.

The other replies were: blood test (15), temperature chart (11), physical examination (10), cervical smear (7), tubal operation (6), laparoscopy (5), fertility drugs (5), uterine scrape (4), hormones (3). Whilst the more common tests and treatments had been quite widely anticipated by some of the patients, there were some surprising results. Few replies mentioned hormones, despite a common concern with this factor. The few references to fertility drugs and operations on the fallopian tubes perhaps would not be replicated now, in view of the enormous increase in the publicity surrounding these developments. Although no record was made of which partner gave which answer, the clear impression was that the bulk of the information came from the woman. It is surprising, perhaps, that the most frequently used treatments or tests were mentioned by only half of the couples.

Overall these replies served to confirm the picture given of their consultations with the GP and discussions with lay contacts. Whether through a failure to absorb the information offered or a lack of information, the couples seemed to be fairly ill-prepared for investigation, in their understanding of the relevant reproductive and fertility facts. Despite a relatively high level of educational attainment, their knowledge of the implications of referral to the Clinic was fairly thin. There was certainly no evidence that a significant number of these couples was motivated by a clear perception of what might be offered by the infertility service. It would be interesting to see the effect of the recent, widespread media attention paid particularly to the more dramatic infertility treatments, on the expectations of couples newly referred.

Throughout this study a recurring theme is the relative impact of childlessness on the man and the woman in a marriage, and its social and emotional effects. With this in mind, the couples were asked: 'If you could choose for the problem to lie with just one of you – which one?' Despite this being a rather extraordinary question to ask in relation to a 'medical' condition, only seven of the men and ten of the women felt unable to make a choice. Of the men making a choice, 14 (61 per cent) wished it to be themselves, the altruistic choice. Amongst the women, 16 (80 per cent) were likewise selfless. Given the common perspective, discussed below, that infertility was experienced more painfully by a woman, it would not have been unreasonable to expect the reverse. The point was made by eight of those 'electing' the woman, that more treatments are available for women than men, as indeed is the case; and more of these treatments are successful.

Various reasons were advanced to explain the choice made, including: the supposed simpler nature of male reproductive processes; greater male/female resilience to the diagnosis of infertility; greater social acceptance of infertility in women. This last point was not put in relation to men. It was clear from the readiness of many of the answers to such a difficult question that, in many cases, it had already been mentally asked. It was clear for many of the couples that they had asked themselves the question 'what if?' more readily than the simpler 'what will happen at the Clinic?'. This was probably an important factor in the unease and anxiety which attended referral to the Clinic for many of the couples in this study.

THE EARLY EFFECTS OF CHILDLESSNESS

The epithet 'early' is not entirely appropriate in the situation already described; these couples had been trying to conceive a child for as long as 11 years before being seen in the Infertility Clinic. However, when they had first contact with the research, they were asked at this earliest point in their specialist treatment what impact they felt childlessness was having on them. At this stage their feelings will be influenced by their circumstances, the reactions of their social circle, and the impact of their encounter with the family GP discussed above. These feelings will not yet have been substantially affected by the process of investigation and the procedures of the Clinic. It is not suggested that the Clinic will have had no effect. As the material already presented makes clear, from the moment of specialist referral being suggested it can be argued that a new, and possibly important, factor enters the situation. In subsequent discussion it may be noted that, not surprisingly, the feelings changed over the period of the research; overall there was a fall in the proportion who felt that childlessness substantially affected them, which was accounted for by those who had a child and seemed then to dismiss the upset of childlessness.

The couples in the study were asked the open-ended question: 'How do you think being childless has affected you so far?' It should be said that only one of those who were asked the question replied that the experience had been positive, and this was severely qualified, and contrasted sharply with the feelings this man expressed at a later stage.

> We quite like the idea of kids, but we're not totally committed. Just want to know one way or the other. We're over 30 now; it has to be in the next year or so, on the borderline then . . . no big deal if we don't . . . not concerned, just a bit worried. (Mrs Keith)

> It's only affected us materially, not mentally at all; we've a tidier house, better standard of living, the wife works. (Mr Keith)

At the final stage of the research, a number of the couples were able to point to positive effects in the experience in relation to the quality of their marriages. The concentration at this stage, however, was on the negative impact that childlessness had on the couple and the way they felt about themselves and each other.

Twenty of the men (67 per cent) felt that they had been affected in some way, and slightly more of the women, 22 (73 per cent). Twenty-four (80 per cent) of the couples had similar feelings about their situation. When these responses were considered, the pattern in Table 5.7 emerged. The striking point is that in no case did the man feel that he suffered stress from the failure to have a child whilst the wife did not. Support was given to this

Table 5.7 Early stress of childlessness

Who felt affected?	No.	%
Neither	6	20
Man only	0	0
Woman only	5	17
Both	19	63

picture in the scores achieved in the self-evaluation questionnaires: the men on average rated themselves as coping better than the women.

Some of the comments made by the couples will illustrate the depth of feeling this experience had created for many of them.

> Rough! The woman suffers more than the man. It's difficult to explain; it's when you see children, people ask when you are going to have them. She's upset, cries a lot. (Mr Green)

The difference between the husband and the wife which typified many of the responses to this question was clearly expressed by the Carters, both teachers.

> Just wish that we could because of the effect that it is having on my wife. Doesn't really affect me, but she's worried and keyed up the whole time. Frustrated, but I don't feel desperate. (Mr Carter)

> Drastically at times; I'm depressed and anxious. It's a severe emotional trauma. It's upset our relationship; I'm crabby, sex isn't always enjoyable, very stressful. (Mrs Carter)

This couple will be discussed further at a later stage. Their marriage did founder during the research period, although there was some disagreement between them as to the relative importance of the childlessness as a cause.

The women expressed their hurt very strongly.

> I'd hate to be told 'you're infertile'; I'd feel half a woman. I get upset seeing people with babies. (Mrs Holt)

> I think not getting pregnant broke up my first marriage; I don't want that to happen again. (Mrs Flower)

> Sometimes I can sit and laugh, but then I start resenting friends, and get very upset, and even start talking to the cat and dog. (Mrs Neal)

> I'm neurotic, a worrier, a whittler [= *worrier, one who frets over trifles*], I get very tense. It worries me that I might not be able to have any, I've left it so long. He's much less bothered. I get down because of it; really fed up about it. I didn't realise I wanted a family as much until we started trying. I feel slightly guilty because of the dieting when I was at college; that led to no periods, losing my hair, not eating properly. I get very upset particularly when someone in the close family has children, I feel very mean and awful, but I feel very jealous; I wish I wasn't. I'd be very upset if my brother or sister had a child. (Mrs Mitchell)

Several persistent themes occur in these comments. Many of the women expressed some of their pain in the form of guilt; one of the reactions to childlessness discussed in Chapter 4. As in the case of Mrs Mitchell, there may be real events in the past of significance for current fertility problems such as over-dieting, or terminations of pregnancy. In both these examples their long-term effects on fertility are not entirely clear. More recent evidence (see Winston 1986) seems to suggest that only in the more severe cases of anorexia is there likely to be subsequent infertility if a recovery is achieved; similarly, particularly as now performed, there is little evidence that properly conducted abortions (TOPs) will impair future fertility. Mrs Mitchell was typical in looking for reasons for her infertility, whereby to blame herself. The medical evidence was that her adolescent dieting was excessive by adult standards but did not amount to severe anorexia. In the same way, she believes she 'has left it so long' and, by implication, decreased the chances of infertility; at the time of referral to the Clinic she was 25, not late on any interpretation of the evidence. Mrs Mitchell was having periods, although not regularly. Her husband proved to have very poor semen, and they achieved pregnancy in the first course of treatment by DI. She put her own history in the worst possible light in the answer quoted above; accepting by implication all the 'blame', without the evidence that the husband might, as proved to be the case, be the principal source of the problem.

This couple also proved to be interesting in that, at the final interview, they firmly stated that their pregnancy was natural, and that the DI had not worked. This was untrue. The couple seemed to have forgotten their agreement that I should have access to their medical notes, and therefore would know their statement almost certainly to be untrue. Naturally I did not challenge them in any way or remind them of my access to the medical notes. It was a clear instance of the trouble a woman will take to collude in keeping the 'secret' of the man's infertility from public knowledge. There were no examples of men taking the same trouble to hide the fertility problems of their wives, other than those cases in which they attempted to release as little information as possible about their problems in general.

The effects of friends and relatives having children was often mentioned, particularly by women. The emotional pain seemed to be caused in three ways, as illustrated in the quotations above. Firstly, these events served as painful reminders of their own problems in failing to conceive a child. These reactions are not dissimilar from the distress associated with the coming of a menstrual period or seeing babies and pregnant women. Many of these women made conscious efforts to avoid the company of expectant women and young children; hence the strong feelings generated by the Infertility Clinic being sited in the Ante-natal Clinic. Secondly, pregnancies, amongst siblings particularly, increased the wondering and questioning by parents and parents-in-law. One of the couples in answering the question 'who is most upset about your difficulty in having a child?'

replied 'grandparents', which they then crossed out and changed to 'parents', i.e. referring to their own parents who deeply wanted to be grandparents. Thirdly, these births caused strong feelings of envy and jealousy, about which they then felt guilt, wanting to feel happiness for the parents concerned, but finding it impossible to separate out their own comparative 'failings'.

Anger was not frequently expressed at this point, although there was much evidence of it later on, often directed at the perceived failings of the Clinic.

> I get upset at the sight of pregnant women, and mothers with lots of children who don't care. It does hurt a lot; though I've not got to the child snatching stage *yet*. The word 'infertility' at the Clinic hurts; it's such a cold word; your last chance.   (Mrs Newsome)

> Why us? we'd give our eye teeth for children, when there's others don't care and batter their kids.   (Mr Newsome)

Stealing babies from their prams was mentioned a number of times in this half-joking manner. The seriousness behind the levity was clear; the couples concerned had little difficulty in empathising with the plight of distraught would-be mothers who resorted to such desperate actions.

Although there was little positive said about the effects of infertility, there were several couples who protested that they were coming to the Clinic in order to find out if there was a medical problem, and whether they were ever likely to be able to have children, and not because they saw themselves as being 'desperate' for children immediately, and at any cost in emotional or physical pain or inconvenience. They challenged the assumption of irrational desperation blamed by Pfeffer and Quick (1988) for the low priority and insensitivity accorded to infertility services. The men took the lead in expressing this position in each case.

> Doesn't worry me, particularly now. Not yearning for children now; but we wouldn't like to think that we'd never have any. Children are a mixed blessing, sacrifices are involved. But if we never have children, I doubt if it'd upset me dreadfully.   (Mr Butler)

> I'd love it to happen, but we've a nice tidy home here, a comfortable rut. It's not the driving force in life. Don't go discussing it a lot. At one time we definitely did not want children. Married quarters (he spent some years in the army) were baby factories, that was awful, we wanted to get set up first. It's no great deal, don't get in a tizz. We're really not bothered, it's just a matter of choice, shall we have our own or adopt?
>   (Mr Keith)

Mr Keith seemed, like Hamlet's mother, to protest too much for his words to be taken at face value. Their persistence over two years in spite of their (particularly his) vehement criticism of the Clinic, its personnel and procedures, tended to contradict this protested lack of real concern.

The effects noted by the Carters have been mentioned already. The other couple, whose marriage collapsed during the course of investigation for infertility, was the Traffords. In quoting their response, in brackets are the notes I made about the verbal and non-verbal process of the interview at the time.

[motioned me to sit on the settee, they then sat either side of me!]

He makes it worse, getting me to watch things on TV about these problems.   (Mrs Trafford)

It's good for you; makes you try harder.   (Mr Trafford)

[she looks away, tears well up]

I get very upset, depressed, tense.   (Mrs Trafford)

Doesn't bother me much.   (Mr Trafford)

[clear differences between them, both confirmed their stated feelings non-verbally, very clearly.]

Another significant strand in the feelings expressed has been mentioned already in respect of the histories of these couples. Where the man had already fathered a child in a previous relationship, so far from reducing the pressure on the woman in the current marriage to 'give him' a child, it appeared, in all the cases in the study, to increase the pressure she felt. Feminist ideas seemed to have had little impact on these couples in the way they described the process of birth in terms of a presentation to the husband. The Traffords were in this position. This feeling was not reflected by the men where the woman already had a child.

It affects me more; most of my friends have children. He's got a child he hardly knows by his first wife. It hurts that I can't give him a child when he loves children so much. I feel resentment, frustration. I get upset over abortion, NAI, things like that. Look on the black side.   (Mrs Ivy)

It's a difficult period to explain at present; the wife's getting upset particularly 'cause I've a child by my first marriage and she wants to give me one.   (Mr Ivy)

In completing the personal questionnaire item comparing their present relationship with when they first married, the men appeared on average to feel slightly less happy than their wives. In rating the attitude of their spouses the majority felt that he or she was very sympathetic. Only seven of both the men and the women (23 per cent) felt that the spouse was either 'quite sympathetic' or 'neutral'. The men were slightly less positive: four felt the spouse was 'neutral' in attitude, compared with only one of the women. At this stage it is notable that none recorded unfavourable verdicts on the spouse's attitude, although they knew that what they had written would not be seen by the partner.

SUMMARY

The evidence is that, for the men and women concerned, seeking medical help is a significant step, not taken lightly. There is substantial delay before the GP is consulted, and, in some cases, even further delay whilst the couple and GP decide whether to take the next step of referral to a specialist.

Whatever the stated practice of GPs in the FPS, the picture emerging of actual practice from the patients at the Clinic is that they are poorly prepared for specialist investigation. They have little information about the process that will be involved; and their level of understanding about the mechanics of reproduction was not impressive. Given the generally positive feelings expressed about the GPs, they might be in a position substantially to smooth the course of infertility investigation and treatment with appropriate medical counselling at this initial stage.

Even at this early stage in their 'careers' as subfertile couples, personal anguish was very evident. Particularly clear was the different experiences and feelings of men and women. The impression was strongly conveyed that pronatalist pressures bore more heavily on the woman. Certain features of the approach of GPs and the Clinic have been mentioned which seem to underscore this differential experience of pressure. Within these early experiences are the seeds of some of the difficulties encountered by these couples as they proceeded with investigation and treatment.

6 Experiencing childlessness

Being childless involves important changes in the way in which couples see themselves, and are seen, both by each other and significant other people in their lives. For childless couples there is no doubt from this study that, to some extent, childlessness involved them in assuming a 'spoiled identity' in the sense discussed by Goffman (1963), which then required active 'management'.

Most of these couples brought to their initial attempts to have children the unquestioning assumption that being healthy and 'normal' was enough to ensure fertility. The only exceptions to this were the couples who had already experienced a fertility-related problem such as menstrual difficulty or had been 'warned' in some way by a previous test or infertile relationship. As will become apparent, such warnings did not necessarily appear to make adjustment to the situation that much easier.

Sutherland vividly expresses the experience of adjusting to such a spoiled identity in relation to physical disability:

> It both depersonalises us and writes us off as individuals by implying that our disabilities are our identity.
>
> (Sutherland 1981: 13)

The concern of this chapter will be to present their experiences of childlessness in the various important arenas.

An overview of their experiences will be presented in this chapter, which illustrates some of the key issues. In a small sample with such differing personal and medical histories the expected diversity of reactions was recorded. It would be potentially misleading to attempt a categorisation of individual patterns of response, where this diversity was compounded with the highly idiosyncratic course each couple trod through the Clinic, each one determined by their own test and treatment results. The picture to be drawn here illustrates some of the more general patterns to be observed in the way couples reacted to the experience of being identified as childless and the investigation that followed.

As might be expected, over time there was some dulling of the recollection of pain associated with childlessness. The comments made concerning the impact of childlessness gave some support to the idea of a process of grief and adjustment, as discussed by Menning (1977) and others, presented in Chapter 2. However, the comments of the Clinic patients will illustrate all of the phases Menning identifies, bearing out the caveat of Murray Parkes (1986) that this process of grief is not a unitary one, through which all individuals move at a predictable pace; rather it is a series of signposts to the important components in their emotional reactions. These ideas proved to have value in understanding the reactions of the couples in this study.

A significant difficulty in using the Murray Parkes' model of grief reaction is that childlessness is not a single event. The 'status' of involuntary childlessness is one that, once identified, is modified over a considerable period of time by the experiences of a variety of medical encounters, various investigative and treatment procedures, and differing outcomes regarding pregnancy. Feelings of hope and optimism were generated by 'good' test results and active treatment of a diagnosed problem, and positive experiences of being understood or helped. Despair and feelings of being bereft could follow the opposite situations, or indeed decisions to redirect their energies.

The grief experienced by childless couples is 'unfocused' as the Houghtons (1977) observe; having no clear object, as would be the case with death or disability. It is the reaction to the failure to achieve something, that is a child, not the loss of something or someone. It is, however, a loss of potential and certain life opportunities, as discussed by Mahlstedt (1985). The reactions received in this enquiry are an existential amalgam of these situations.

The concern of this chapter is to consider the experiences of the childless couples. Childlessness was not an isolated event for many of these people, but a lengthy period of considerable distress causing some detailed personal review of themselves and their important relationships.

PERSONAL IMPACT OF CHILDLESSNESS

The nature and extent of the impact of the experience of infertility and childlessness on the couples in this study varied considerably. I shall concentrate on their perceptions of these effects.

Personal distress

There was a striking difference in the extent to which men and women admitted to feeling upset about their childlessness. Initially they seemed to have similar feelings, but the men apparently became less likely to say they were upset, whilst the women increasingly admitted to being upset.

The obvious difficulty in interpreting this finding is that it only measures the willingness in an interview to admit to feeling upset or worried about the situation. In turn this is naturally affected by the role model internalised by each respondent of the feelings which he or she believes is regarded as appropriate to one in that position. The discussion of pronatalism and attitudes to parenting relates to these perceptions. Social expectations, it was suggested, emphasise that motherhood is of pre-eminent importance to a woman, whereas for men fatherhood is but one of a range of life goals which is not necessarily of greater significance than, say, career or income or social achievement. It is also the case that it is more acceptable in our society for women to express feelings of hurt or anxiety, and discuss emotions, than is the case for men.

Table 6.1 conceals a substantial degree of individual variation over the period of the study, however. All the possible combinations of responses to these questions about being worried or upset were given. Only five (20 per cent) of the men answered affirmatively at every stage of the study, compared with 21 (70 per cent) of the women. In each of these five cases, the woman also, at each stage, said that she was upset. In the other 16 cases in which at every stage the woman said she was upset, the husband gave a variety of responses. This suggests that the man's consistent admission of being upset was only experienced or admitted when the wife shared the feelings. The reverse was not true. Only five (17 per cent) of the husbands denied feeling upset at every stage, and three (10 per cent) of the wives.

A significant pattern concerns the reactions of the men interviewed. There was a marked fall in the numbers of those who said that they were worried or upset, whilst the numbers of women remained fairly constant. It might be the case that these feelings of upset were more likely to be openly admitted where the childlessness was subsequently overcome. Of the five men who admitted to feeling upset on each occasion they were interviewed, only one remained childless at the end of the study; nine of the 21 women

Table 6.1 Admitted worry/upset

	I [1]	%	*FU1* [2]	%	*FU2* [3]	%
Men	19	63	13	43	13	43
Women	24	80	25	83	25	83

1. Initial interview
2. First follow-up interview
3. Second follow-up interview

in this position remained without children. The differences were not so much between those whose childlessness was successfully remedied and those who remained without children, as between men and women.

Women in this study appeared to be more ready to express feelings of worry and upset over their experiences of childlessness than the men. The impressions of conducting the interviews and other evidence presented below, suggested that the women were indeed more likely to be upset. In addition, there was some evidence that the feelings of the man were less likely to be dependent on those of his wife; that is, where the man admitted feeling upset the woman almost invariably expressed the same feelings, but the man did not reflect the feelings of his wife to anything like the same degree.

How, then, did these men and women describe the effect of their difficulty in having children, and the experience of attending the Infertility Clinic? The women most articulated feeling upset.

> I used to get so desperate, every month, it was a dreadful time . . . I was very jealous of other women who were pregnant. I could never settle to anything. Now (we have had a child) we're thinking of going to the Channel Isles for a holiday; then it was always thinking of having a baby. Made me very bitter – not bitter – towards women who were pregnant – very resentful. Made me pretty miserable. When my sister was pregnant, I sobbed my heart out. I was quite obsessed with it. It became my whole life, thinking about it the whole time.   (Mrs Quick)

This quotation illustrates some of the typical components in this emotional upset, which were discussed in relation to comments made when they were first interviewed (see Chapter 5); the personal pain as well as the resentment over the success of others. This jealousy or resentment emerged as one of the worrying features for them of the personal reaction to their situation. In every case that this arose, the woman – as in the case of Mrs Quick – was appalled at feeling the way she did. Added to the envy, then, was the guilt of experiencing such feelings; particularly, as was the case so often, when the object of these strong feelings was a close relative or friend.

The extent of the preoccupation was often expressed.

> I got unbearable to live with . . . I was really miserable a lot of the time. You hardly ever saw me with a smile on my face . . . just got really depressed when going through the infertility thing. I used to cry and cry, anything would set me off.   (Mrs Newsome)

> I couldn't sleep at night, I couldn't eat. It really depresses you. I just felt like going away . . . I asked myself 'what am I living for?'   (Mrs Holt)

I feel like I'm in limbo; I know what I want, I want kids, but I can't ever see me having them. I'm a pessimist; I don't know what I'll do if I never have them. (Mrs Neal)

Few of the women claimed not to have been affected, as already indicated. Those who did had little to add to the denial. Mrs Underwood, who was unable to have children, put this minority position succinctly:

Don't think it has; some are more desperate to have children than others. Nothing comes to mind; I feel no different. I felt sorry for Dan [sterile] but it made no difference.

The men in the study were, as already indicated, much more likely to claim not to have been upset by the experience.

I never remember being worried about it; I'm not well up in the biological ins and outs of it. I didn't feel anxiety about it in the family sense that Ellen did . . . She felt really jealous when my sister had a child, which I did not feel at all. (Mr Carter)

No. Quite easy either way. It wouldn't have affected me either way.
(Mr Butler)

It hasn't really, I'm a realist, if people say 'no' I'll accept no. Not bothered by the actual saying we can't have children, no.
(Mr Trafford)

On the self-evaluation questionnaires, which were checked and rated by the partner, the men scored themselves as being more extrovert than the women, less neurotic, and more coping. In addition, those who admitted being upset did indeed, on average, score as more neurotic, less extrovert and less coping than those who claimed not to be upset by the experience.

When the partner was asked to 'mark' the other's self-assessment it seemed that the couples were less likely to disagree with their spouse's assessment of these personality characteristics at the later stage, whether or not they had children in the interim.

This must be interpreted with some care; however, it might be reasonable to suggest that this is also support for the impression that one of the effects of the experience of childlessness is that marriages which remain intact show a higher level of mutual understanding than previously, not the increased distance that has been predicted.

The evidence of these questionnaires appears to support the finding that not only are the men less upset in the beginning by their childlessness, as they say themselves, but they become less upset over time, whether or not the childlessness is resolved successfully. The personal hurt for the women remains, even if they are able to have a child; if they fail to have a child this becomes markedly worse.

There was some evidence that a diagnosis of infertility may have a negative impact on the individual's feelings of being able to cope with ordinary social obligations. It suggested that such a diagnosis is particularly significant for feeling able to cope amongst the women affected.

Depression

The couples were specifically asked if they ever got fed up or depressed, and whether or not they felt this bore any relation to their experience of childlessness. Amongst the men, ten (37 per cent) had noticed a change in their experience of depression (in this non-technical sense); the five who felt they were in general less depressed than they used to be were all parents by this time, whereas the five who felt more depressed remained childless, although it has to be said that only three of these men linked this change to infertility. A similar pattern appeared amongst the women; 19 (68 per cent) remarked on a change in their general mood over this period, ten feeling less depressed, all of whom were now mothers, and nine feeling more depressed, eight of whom were childless. (The one woman not fitting this trend was experiencing family illnesses at the time of the interview.) None of the men had sought advice for these feelings. Three of the women had mentioned these feelings to their GPs. Mrs Newsome and Mrs Neal had been prescribed tranquillisers, although Mrs Newsome had resisted taking them. Mrs Lamb had more difficulty coping on her own, although she felt that the infertility was very much exacerbated by the fact of her husband being away so much. In order to get employment, he had to take a job which required him to live away from home for part of the week.

> A couple of years ago I got panic attacks and daren't go out. I got really depressed then. I think that was because of being left on my own. Mick was working in London for two years. Still get these a little, but don't feel that they've got much to do with the infertility. I was stuck in the house a lot, it would be much better if I'd got work. The doctor gave me tranquillisers, but I went back no different, and he referred me to a psychiatrist. He knew everything I was going through, complete insecurity, no confidence in myself. I went two or three times, he gave me a relaxation tape; that's one of the problems, I can't relax . . . The GP just said 'do your hands shake? then take these tranx'; I just needed someone to say 'No, you're not going mad'.

Mr Lamb felt that these problems were in fact very much to do with the infertility. It was clear that Mr Lamb's finding work locally had not resolved the situation entirely. This woman's predicament also illustrates a dilemma referred to already. It is one of the common folk remedies for infertility that the woman should stop working. Whilst this might have a beneficial effect on her physical and emotional stress level, thus aiding conception (although there is little evidence to support this view, as discussed in Chapter 2), it does have the secondary effect of increasing the preoccupation with conceiving a child due to the removal of other outlets and interests, and possibly increasing the general sense of isolation.

None of the men interviewed reported any nervous problems in connection with their experience of infertility, although seven women did, five of whom had not been able to conceive. Mrs Lamb, Mrs Neal and those who suffered from post-natal depression – Mrs Carver, Mrs Newsome and Mrs Quick (discussed in Chapter 8 in relation to relationships with the children who were born after a period of infertility) – were the only ones to have consulted their GPs for help with psychological problems. Mrs Crow, who remained childless, had been investigated for loss of sensation in her facial muscles which was tentatively diagnosed by a dermatologist as psychological in origin, although treatment was not considered. Mrs Holt reported that:

> It's been a lot worse since the [unsuccessful] operation; I've been getting depressed each month, but I've not been to the doctor.

Mrs Trafford spoke of 'just sitting, breaking down, crying. But even that's better than just thinking about it.' 'I witter – worry about Karen [daughter], but not like before' was how Mrs Mitchell put it on reflection. Several of the women who had been able to conceive made this clear distinction between their current feelings and how they remembered being whilst trying to get pregnant.

The sense of shock and pain was vividly expressed by Mrs Newsome on hearing that the results of tests had been poor:

> Felt shocked, hurt, why us? took some sinking in. Rough going having to accept it . . . feel right [= *really*] isolated even at the Clinic or in the hospital; it would be nice to talk to others in the same boat and compare feelings, you don't know how others feel. Feel very hurt deep down . . . and alone; everyone else can have them, always see people on the telly with their bellies stuck out. I'm really sensitive to so many people getting pregnant; makes it doubly worse.

She also put the feelings of being so much alone quite clearly in this comment, echoed by Mrs Mitchell:

> I felt a bit of a failure. The name 'infertility clinic' felt a bit of a let down,

awful; like being called barren. You do feel very isolated . . . think the world is against me. What have I done wrong?

The role played by others in reinforcing this sense of isolation by their silence was expressed by Mrs Urmston:

One of the troubles is people don't talk about it. Like when I had the miscarriage, my neighbour came in to see me when I got back from the hospital. [Afterwards I found out] they'd all said to her 'now don't say anything, she'll be upset'. But I was never upset because they said anything, just like the infertility; I felt much better when she'd talked to me about it.

Others saw one of the positive aspects of attending the Clinic as bringing home the reality that infertility is a problem faced by many people.

Feel less on our own seeing others there.   (Mrs Turner)

You think there's only you, then you realise how many there is.

(Mrs David)

Following up these women over a substantial period demonstrated the healing of these feelings of hurt which occurred over time. Mrs Holt, in our last interview, expressed this move towards resignation and acceptance predicted by the model of bereavement:

I just feel numb now. First few months I couldn't sleep at night. I couldn't eat. It really depresses you, I just felt like going away . . . The feelings have lasted a long time: really bad when I was just out of hospital [for laparo-scopy]. I was so tired but I couldn't sleep; but I haven't been quite so bad recently; I've been thinking there's people a lot worse off than you. I know there's nothing I can do. I still think 'why'd it happen?'

The importance of reaching some conclusion and firm diagnosis in permitting this process to occur satisfactorily was demonstrated in the comments of Mrs Young. The parallel can be made with those people discussed by Murray Parkes (1986) who lose someone in an accident or as a result of crime without the body being recovered; they seem to have particular difficulty in coming to terms with the death. The Youngs had withdrawn at an early stage of investigation without hearing the results of the tests.

I feel all mixed up, me. I've got very aggressive . . . something goes wrong and I'll just fly. I seem all confused about it. He thinks I'm stupid ['yes'-Mr] . . . can't explain to him, feel all muddled up about it . . . I do want family, but it confuses me; if I knew the results it would help.

This couple had failed two appointments to hear the results of tests. During the time of the study they did not make a further appointment, although being given details of how to achieve this if they wished. In her case, the fear of finding out that there was a serious problem which would forever make conception impossible was greater than the anxiety of continuing not to conceive as she and her husband so much wanted. It did seem to be postponing the time when they might resolve their situation.

Husbands' and wives' views of each others' reactions

The wives, asked at first follow-up what impact childlessness had made on their husbands, said 'none' twice as often as their husbands when asked the same question concerning their wives (13:7), confirming the husband's own view in most cases.

In one case, the explanation for the failure to be upset was that he had 'not felt the involved party'. This was the case in which the husband, Mr Mitchell, had severe oligospermia and they conceived a child through DI, which they subsequently denied to me. This denial of concern could there-fore have been part of the same elaborate smoke-screen. In itself, this strategy suggested strong feelings on his part with which either he or they were unable or unwilling to come to terms. In one case, it was clear that the wife did not expect the husband to be prepared to become involved at all.

> I admire him for going to hospital for investigation at all: didn't think he would! (Mrs Underwood)

The Urmstons were a particularly striking case in which the wife appeared to carry all the burden of their failure to have children right up to the point at which the husband was diagnosed subfertile. In both earlier interviews, Mr Urmston had denied feeling upset about their problems, at which time his position had not been finally adjudicated.

Mr Neal expressed vividly the feeling that what made the experience most upsetting was the effect it had on his wife.

> I felt she was cracking up, going without sleep, dreaming during the day, nervous all the time, wanting to sleep all the time; the periods were still coming all the time though. (Mr Neal)

> Only affects him when I get upset, and start driving him nuts. (Mrs Neal)

In accepting their feelings of hurt, many of the men noted that their wives had suffered more than they had.

> Didn't bother me the same as Delia. (Mr Trafford)

It was always more important to Josie, I wasn't really all that bothered. Women seem to want children more. I was more interested in cars before we had her. Josie *really* wanted children, I just went along with it. It wasn't until Debbie was born I got so involved. It's after they're born with men.　　　　　　　　　　　　　　　　　　　　　(Mr Diamond)

It gets to you, but don't think it affects you as much as the woman. Felt you were missing out on something. I used to think about it but not a person to get depressed; I bottle it up. Thought about it a lot.
　　　　　　　　　　　　　　　　　　　　　　　　　　　(Mr Thurston)

Issue of virility

Some of the husbands said that they had been upset by the experience, and some admitted to having been depressed, as has been illustrated already. However, most responses to this question were in relation to the investigations or diagnosis made (where it had been one of male infertility) or in relation to the effect of the upset on the wife.

Upsetting; feels like a corridor of doors shutting in front of you.
　　　　　　　　　　　　　　　　　　　　　　　　　　　　(Mr Green)

Felt that the referral happened so quickly, shocked at the speed; pushed into doing something too quickly; children aren't the be-all and end-all.
　　　　　　　　　　　　　　　　　　　　　　　　　　　(Mr Truswell)

Criticism of the Clinic was particularly expressed by the husbands, as will be seen from the next chapter. This seemed to be the focus by which the men interviewed felt able to express their feelings about infertility.

I was more upset at the news of the sperm problem than I care to admit; and hurt at feeling hurt. Don't know how other men cope. The he-man, macho image takes a bit of a knock . . . It got to me, changed me, made me less brash. It really dented my self confidence . . . it's been like living under a cloud; it's been hard . . . I turned all the anger in on myself.
　　　　　　　　　　　　　　　　　　　　　　　　　　　(Mr Truswell)

He's been very quiet too, he hasn't said much; a bit bitter they can't do anything for him; no drugs, nothing!　　　　　　　　　　　(Mrs Green)

The perception of male infertility as automatically impugning virility was keenly felt by a number of the men in this study. The stigma of infertility for men relates closely to the prevalence of this 'folk belief', that fertility and virility are inseparable. Ethologists could point to many examples amongst mammals where behavioural evidence does indicate that these two characteristics are indeed often closely linked (e.g. Lorenz 1963), which might point to some important atavistic trait in man. No association has so far been demonstrated in human sexual behaviour. It was striking that the only counterpart amongst the women was the feeling of failing the husband; not a sense of being less feminine. This is a comparison that Pfeffer and Woollett (1983) make much of in their discussion of the impact of infertility; causing Newill in a review in *NACK* magazine (1984) unfairly to castigate them for their 'negative view of men'. Without this being true in all cases, there was clearly a tendency amongst several of the husbands to respond emotionally to the diagnosis of infertility in terms of a perception of themselves as men.

> Felt numb for quite a few days, because of the shock. We didn't expect I'd have problems, as I've got a kid already. It's a weird experience. Got over it over time, but it's still there. Suddenly all the TV and papers are full of test-tube babies and children in care. Can't put it out of your mind. It seems to be pushed. Soon as it involves you, it hits you, and people seem to be asking suddenly. We've not told anyone, not even her parents; no point in worrying them . . . Afraid of people joking about it; you can't expect much sympathy.   (Mr Urmston)

The effects of previous parenthood

All of the men who had children in previous relationships saw that as reducing their concern about having children with their wife.

> Having two children already obviously makes it less distressing for me than Hannah. It makes me irritable when she is upset. She's so impatient, can't get it out of her mind.   (Mr Flower)

It was noticeable that the only woman (Mrs Holt) who had already had a child in another partnership did not feel that this in any way reduced the feeling of failure and hurt.

In other instances, the husband expressed his hurt as anger towards the Clinic.

> It's never off your mind; it gets out of all proportion. She's been doing her temperature chart every day for 3½ years; not surprising it gets her down . . . I'm a very intolerant individual who expects results not excuses. I get very annoyed and upset when anyone upsets Jenny. I'm a getter of things done, so it's very frustrating for me. It's the frustration of not having the choice.   (Mr Crow)

Sense of isolation

The couples were asked questions intended to elicit the extent to which they were prepared to discuss their fertility problems and treatment with significant people in their social network. On the first occasion four (13 per cent) women and 14 (47 per cent) men had told no one about the Clinic appointment. At the second follow-up these numbers fell to two (7 per cent) women and seven (23 per cent) men.

The other measure of withholding information about their childlessness was obtained by answers to questions concerning the attitudes of family, friends and colleagues or workmates. (At initial interview three wives felt the question concerning colleagues did not apply as they were 'housewives'; at second follow-up all felt able to reply in relation to colleagues they had during the period of their infertility, although in many cases by this time not employed outside the home. All the unemployed men felt able to answer, having been in employment at some time during this period.)

Table 6.2 indicates how many of the respondents believed that their fertility problems were not known to the different key parts of their social networks. At each stage the men were less likely to have confided in each of these groups, and, overall, had confided less widely. It is also clear that the circle of those given the information did widen over time, as might be expected. The only clear exceptions to this were the three couples who conceived through DI, all of whom intended telling as few people as possible the circumstances of their babies' conceptions.

These responses seem to confirm the research finding of gender differences in intimate behaviour: in our society men are socialised to be less open than women in confiding personal matters to others. Ryan (1985) and Richards (1982) outline the way in which male socialisation devalues and discourages the expression of feeling. Brearley (1986) believes that men tend to be more cut off from their feelings. The subject of infertility seemed to offer a clear example of this.

Table 6.2 Social networks which 'do not know'

		Friends	Family	Workmates	Total
Men	I	11	9	17	37
	FU2	9	4	14	27
Women	I	8	6	9	23
	FU2	4	3	8	15

We're both very keen on children, and we do get upset talking about the problems, seeing programmes about kids in need or abused, on telly, or visiting relatives with new babies. We both weep easily. Haven't discussed this with anyone except you. (Mr Young)

Summary

The lasting impression of these interviews is of deep and lasting hurt expressed by many couples, although not all, at the experience of childlessness. This was more strongly expressed as personal pain by the women, whilst the men more often expressed their feelings in relation to their wives, their own diagnosis or the process of investigation. There was evidence that the upset diminished over time, but was not obliterated, even by the birth of children. Many of the reactions suggested that the analogy with bereavement is a helpful one, in that the same feelings were clearly illustrated, although not as a unitary process. In considering the provision of services to childless people, it is important that these feelings are recognised, together with their sense of isolation in not being able to share feelings of hurt or failure.

CHILDLESSNESS AND THE MARRIAGE

The research evidence discussed in Chapter 2 is inconclusive concerning the likely impact of infertility and its treatment on the marital relationship of affected couples. The longitudinal design of this study offered an opportunity to look at this impact on these couples attending the Infertility Clinic. Several sets of information are available on this question.

Perceptions of the marriage

At first and final interview the couples were asked to rate their relationship in comparison with when they first married (Table 6.3). This was asked via the self-evaluation questionnaire, which was handed straight back to me. The main impression of these answers is that, with the exception of the two couples who separated during the study, little disenchantment with the marriage was registered and there was on average little change during the study.

For the purposes of computer analysis the initial and follow-up scores were aggregated and tests run for any associations. There did appear to be an association between these mean scores and whether or not the childlessness was remedied (Table 6.4). Treating the data in this way suggested that those remaining childless felt rather less positive about their

Table 6.3 Perception of marriage: 1

		Mean	Max.	Min.
Man	I	1.92	3.4	1
	FU2	2	3	1
Woman	I	1.83	3.8	1
	FU2	1.99	3	1

1 = substantial improvement; 3 = no change; 5 = substantial deterioration

Table 6.4 Perception of marriage: 2

	Man	*Woman*
Parent	3.45	3.41
Childless	4.52	4.31

2 = substantial improvement; 6 = no change; 10 = substantial deterioration

Man: *T*=-1.90, *P*=0.07; Woman: *T*=-1.66, *P*=0.11.

marriages than did those who had a child. However, this association did not attain statistical significance. Questions of this sort are open to the interpretation that 'no change' is the appropriate answer if the respondent feels that the marriage has always been strong. The judgement 'no change' might in these circumstances be entirely positive.

On the same questionnaire, however, respondents were asked to rate the attitude of their spouse to the difficulties. Not surprisingly, 77 per cent consistently rated their spouse as 'very sympathetic' and none as less than 'neutral'. The ratings as less than 'very sympathetic' came disproportionately from those who remained childless; 65 per cent rather than 46 per cent. This seems to suggest, despite the above finding, that some diminution in the level of satisfaction with the marriage may have occurred. These findings must be treated with great caution for the reasons previously stated, and set alongside the following results from the interviews.

Views of the marriage

When the couples were asked in the interview for their views of the overall changes in their marriage during the period which included investigation for infertility, a more positive picture emerged. Fourteen of the couples (47 per cent) claimed that the relationship was closer. Five (17 per cent) expressed diverging views, all of which involved one partner feeling the marriage had not been affected whilst the other felt that it was closer; in all but one of these cases it was the wife who believed that the relationship had become closer; seven (23 per cent) felt that their marriage was just the same and unaffected; in every case this was said as a measure of satisfaction that the marriage was already sound.

Four couples (13 per cent), two of whom had separated, felt the marriage had suffered, all of whom remained childless at the final interview. Ten of the 14 couples (71 per cent) who felt the marriage had become closer were by this time parents, and only four (29 per cent) were still childless, which might suggest some negative impact of childlessness on the marriage.

Almost half of the couples interviewed claimed that their marriage had been cemented by the experiences of childlessness and investigation at the hospital Clinic.

> It's brought us closer; we were close anyway. He's very supportive, but I still felt a bit on my own. Sometimes I'd say 'get yourself another woman who can have a baby for you'. I'd take it out on him and reject him. It is hard to cope with. It's not sympathy so much as someone to share the problems you need; he's pulled me out of it. If I'd been younger I might have left him. (Mrs Newsome)

It is interesting to compare this reaction with that reported above by men faced with a diagnosis of sterility. It was noted there that the distress experienced by men was particularly likely to be expressed in relation to a poor prognosis. The difference amongst the women was striking. Feelings of 'not being a proper woman' were expressed only by Mrs Holt, who quickly went on to explain this in terms of it representing a failure to fulfil the wife's 'duty' of giving her husband a child. It seemed to be acceptable for the men not to explain their feelings as much in terms of a duty to their wife. Three women had at some time told their husbands that the failure to conceive would justify the latter ending the marriage. This was another indication that the burden of childlessness appears to fall disproportionately on the woman.

> It made us talk more and be more aware of each other's feelings. At first I thought he didn't mind really. He doesn't show his feelings much, but I learned just how much he really does feel – that same weekend he was really heart-broken [when after 40 days her period came]. It brought us closer. (Mrs Coleman)

The extent to which the man was able to share his feelings was a recurring theme in these answers. It was several times stated that a significant element in the relationship becoming closer was, contrary to usual practice, the husband expressing his emotional pain openly to his wife. The counterpart to this situation was observed (as much as heard) in the replies of Mr and Mrs Mitchell:

> He upsets me sometimes, he's so laid back about it, not intense like I am. He's the eternal optimist and I'm the eternal pessimist.

> She's better than when you came last!

> [JHM noted: 'his laid-backness clearly irritates her a lot!']

Although they claimed to feel closer since the period of infertility, now resolved, it was apparent that the extent to which feelings are openly shared remained an unresolved issue.

> It brought us closer together. Now we tend not to bother about small problems. We're a lot more tolerant of each other. Everything is shared. It makes you grow up fast; more tolerant of other people too, and we listen to each other better.   (Mr Quick)

> Whole infertility thing, then the investigations, then having him [their son] and the depression, brought us closer together. We're much closer friends than when we were first married.   (Mrs Quick)

The Quicks typically saw this experience as a crisis in their marriage. In most respects, other than the time limits, this fits the classical model of a crisis as described by Caplan (1961). Within the longer term disruption, certain crisis peaks were apparent, e.g. diagnosis, delayed periods. The experience is seen as a major threat to basic needs with which their habitual problem-solving strategies cannot cope – the pressure to 'grow up'. In the sense in which it is used in medicine, the crisis was perceived as a situation of disequilibrium, a turning point, from which the pattern of the marriage would take its future course, 'for better or worse' – 'we tend not to bother about small problems . . .more tolerant'. In coping with this disruption the couple learned better coping strategies – 'listen better . . . closer friends'.

Avoiding the attribution of blame is clearly of considerable importance. Many couples seemed to find it hard to select their words when describing the source of the fertility problem. Those books written for infertile couples (e.g. Newill 1974, Jones 1991) stress the dangers of seeing the partner with the identified impairment as 'to blame' or 'guilty' or even 'responsible' – carrying, as these words seem to, the implication that infertility is a problem for an individual rather than the couple. Blame is, not surprisingly, seen in the literature to be an unsound basis for a marriage. Several couples recognised this explicitly:

At the beginning we agreed never to start blaming the other one. Made a pact such as that and we've stuck to it. We've never pointed the finger, saying it's your fault. (Mr Trevor)

Never thought 'Roy can't have children, I'm going to take it out on him'. We've helped each other through it. (Mrs Trevor)

In the previous chapter it was noted that the need to avoid blame led one couple to deny completely the reality of the husband's infertility (Mitchells). The only exception to this sensitivity was the Grindrods, the couple who had never enjoyed a normal sex life due to the extreme distaste for sexual intercourse felt by Mrs Grindrod.

I do see him as less of a man sometimes, I've got to admit it; it's awful to think that isn't it? But I only say it when I'm angry, but he's so placid, he just takes it.

Yet despite these attitudes – their failure to conceive a child and their continuing, almost non-existent sex life – there was no evidence that this marriage was in difficulty. Both described the relationship as unaffected, as good as when they first married. Nor was there any other sign of marital difficulty. Mr Grindrod accepted such negative statements as placidly as he was described.

The relative importance of the infertility experience was not always clear to the couple who judged their relationship to be closer. The Lambs express it well for many of these couples when they use the metaphor of a common goal.

Since we've been involved it's brought us closer together; given us a common goal. Anyway we've lived so long together, we've mellowed together. (Mr Lamb)

We are much closer together, but it may not be anything to do with the infertility. Don't think it's affected us that much really. Made us discuss things more; it began with the Clinic, perhaps we then got on to talking about other things. (Mrs Lamb)

The Neals speak for those who felt that their relationship had actually prospered under the pressure of infertility and hospital investigation. They highlighted the process of mutual accommodation, or moving towards each other, that many couples described, and also the gradual finding of perspective within which to view the problems. As already pointed out, most of the couples in this position had become parents, just as had the Neals.

I don't know: I think Roger could appreciate me more. Other people don't understand what it was all like. I felt sorry for him – blokes used to make jokes about it. It depended how I felt, how I'd react. Sometimes I could hit them, other times I wasn't bothered. Now we can look back and see other people have worse problems. The ginormous load is lifted off you, but if you went back, you'd still feel it. Only now can I get it straight.   (Mrs Neal)

Had us moments of joy when they said they'd found the cause of the problem and could treat it. I always went with her; it was a joint thing. It was our problem, and we went through it together.   (Mr Neal)

To begin with it was a helluva strain; we really had to know each other. People can live together and not really know each other, but something as intimate as infertility, you really have to get to know each other.
                                                                                    (Mrs Neal)

Almost a quarter of the couples felt that their marriage had not been substantially affected by the experience of infertility. Most, like the Dorairajes and the Underwoods, both of whom were still childless, were keen to say that they had 'always been close' and were 'still happy'. There was no suggestion from any of these couples that 'not affected' might have meant 'no better'.

No effect on our marriage – have freedom in our marriage, each goes where we want, not tied down to one another . . . don't believe anyone who says it has no effect . . . just depends on life style you have. Some can but don't want them.   (Mr Underwood)

No, felt we were always happy; but looking back, perhaps you were more anxious than I thought at the time. You were probably trying to play it down.   (Mr Butler)

No, having gone through the experience we would have accepted it. I'd have sacrificed more than him . . . It was a strong marriage anyway. In some ways it was flattering, he was satisfied with me as I was, not just so that I could provide him with a child.   (Mrs Butler)

This couple were successful in having a child. Again there arose the unquestioned assumption that the wife failing to give the husband a child was of more significance than the reciprocal position. With no abnormality found there could have been a problem on either side. Mrs Butler, having already had a terminated pregnancy, might have suggested the likelihood of difficulties on his side. Mrs Butler claimed to have told her husband of the premarital abortion of another man's child, but asked that it not be raised with him again. From their non-verbal behaviour there was every indication that this was indeed an affectionate and sound marriage.

Husband and wife did not necessarily agree in their assessment of the effects of this experience on their marriage. All but one of the disagreements were in the direction of the husband disclaiming a positive effect noted by the wife. The Truswells were categorised as the couple where the husband more than his wife felt they had become closer. As can be seen, they are not far from agreeing that they have become closer.

A bit closer than other couples who've just decided not to have children. We've been through a lot together. Hard to know. Don't know if we are closer or just that we feel we ought to be. Don't know how close we'd be anyway . . . There was an unsettled patch around the time of getting the news from [the hospital], getting unsure what to say.

(Mrs Truswell)

I think it made us sit down earlier than other people and deliberately plan things . . . We got married for life . . . we work at it . . . Only 18 months married when we went to [the Clinic], but infertility not the only factor – also getting older, longer married . . . Certainly closer but what percentage I don't know. Other people tell us we look close, seem happily married. (Mr Truswell)

The Newsomes also described their experience as very difficult for the marriage, with Mrs Newsome feeling they had finally reached a stronger position than previously. Once again they are close to agreeing that overall the marriage was stronger.

Our marriage was nearly on the rocks at one time. I felt it was all too much. But we were able to talk to each other, and that saved us. I used to get really ratty with him . . . I'd be rotten to Norman; 'you go and find someone who can give you a child'. You say some awful things, and you want to hurt the nearest one to you. After two or three years of going through it we came very close to splitting up. We gave up the flat; everything was getting on top of me. We'd gone so far, everything semt [= *seemed*] to pile on top. The infertility made everything else worse. When I got caught [= *pregnant*], the marriage was still shaky, and I wasn't sure what would happen. But it made all the difference; we was lucky really.

(Mrs Newsome)

You've no chance if the marriage is shaky when you start. When we were going through it the slightest thing could upset the wife. If you really care you can't argue back as you'd normally do. You've got to be careful over everything you say. (Mr Newsome)

This couple had only recently given birth to the long-awaited child. There seemed little doubt in their minds that the crisis of infertility had been resolved and would probably lead to a stronger marriage in the future. The uncertainty appeared to reflect the newness of their parenthood more than fundamental doubts over the relationship.

Finally there were the four couples, still childless, who felt that overall the experience had been deleterious for their marriage.

The mildest of these situations was that of Mr and Mrs Young. The consensus of their views was arrived at only after some discussion in the interview. Mrs Young initially seemed to be offended at her husband's judgement that they were less close as a couple as a result of the infertility. The illustration that he insisted supported his position related to a club to which they had both belonged for some time, but which he felt he was now being edged away from by his wife and her friends. 'I get left out of things more; we're not closer.' They clearly had not discussed this perception before, and the controversy continued for a quarter of an hour before they offered the consensus that, perhaps, things were not quite as easy, but both were adamant that it was more a change in the nature of the relationship than any weakening of it. There was no other evidence of fragility in the marriage.

The Holts were the only couple not to be legally married, and it became clear that their failure to have a child was firmly associated in their minds with the failure to marry, as had been their stated intention at the first interview. Mrs Holt also felt the 'responsibility' not to deny her partner the chance of children. Marriage 'would not be fair to Manny'. A full understanding of this situation was hard to achieve with Mr Holt being deaf and dumb. Communication between them presented no problem for ordinary discourse, but it was plain that issues of feeling and emotion were not easily managed. Neither was able to use sign language fluently, and it also seemed that they were not used to communicating about feelings. Mrs Holt had to act as interpreter for her husband who was in all the interviews very passive, giving only minimal replies to the questions. At the final interview, Mrs Holt painted a bleak picture of the relationship, saying they didn't talk about anything much, 'little contact altogether'. Mrs Holt said to me, which he would not have 'heard' as he was looking away at the time, 'I don't think there's a lot of future in it [the relationship]', although she also seemed to be hoping that things would change if she did become pregnant. Sadly for them, soon after this last interview they received a letter from the hospital removing her from the IVF programme waiting list on the basis of a number of factors, including their unmarried status.

> For a while I was rejecting him; I told Helen [her daughter] 'don't bring him in [to the hospital at the time of the laparoscopy], I don't want to see him again'. But then I began to see it's not fair. But I still felt that resentment, as though I was blaming him. Don't know why; from the

start he was keener than me to have a baby . . . Drawn away more or less. I keep putting off getting married as I still don't know if I can have children . . . He never expresses his feelings: much of the time I don't want to be bothered speaking to him.

It was hard to see much future in this relationship, in the circumstances in which they were soon to find themselves, i.e. permanent childlessness. In this case infertility seemed to be the key factor; if the relationship did end, it would have been largely the result of this 'failure', as Mrs Holt described it.

Two couples actually separated during the course of the study, but in rather different circumstances. The role of childlessness was clearly much more central in the case of the Traffords.

Mr Trafford had been married before and had a teenage daughter, Jackie, by that marriage, who latterly had come to live with them. He was older than his wife, who expressed strongly the feelings that she needed to be able to give him a child, or be diminished as a woman in his eyes. As noted above (p. 107) the strains were apparent early on, but the decision to separate was made only in the week of my final visit. I was able to interview them both, as they were still living in the same house intermittently; although I interviewed them on separate evenings. The attitude of Mr Trafford to his wife's feelings may be judged from the following comments.

She was so upset about not getting pregnant, it soured her relationship with Jackie. I started spending more time out of the house, and that caused more rows . . . Not having children is a big thing for her; she's always wanted one. It's the be-all and end-all for her. It's really jealousy at back of it. She's jealous of me for having Jackie already; that's why it all happened. She got on well with her to start with; then, not long after we married, we tried, and nothing happened. That's when she turned against her. No hatred or owt [= *anything*], she just can't accept it. Probably at first I over-reacted; I fought back for Jackie, and things got worse and worse . . . The investigation gave us hope in a way. But last time he said there's only 5 per cent chance or test-tube. That didn't help . . . It did affect my feelings, because I knew deep down, I knew Delia desperately wanted a child. I couldn't understand why she couldn't be the same with Jackie as she'd been before we got married . . . I wanted a child by Delia; I suggested it. I never said 'I've got one, I don't want anymore'. She's never come out and said 'You don't know how I feel'.

Mr Trafford had played the minimal part in the process of investigation required of him by the Clinic. There was no sense that he owned the problem as a shared responsibility, although both appeared to have impaired fertility, notwithstanding his fatherhood. His sperm was of borderline quality; but he failed to keep appointments for the prescribed hormonal test; he dropped out after receiving the doubtful result, although his wife continued to attend for some months.

Mrs Trafford's view of the situation was rather different to the one her husband painted.

> He never understood what I was going through, or even tried to. This started rows over other things . . . I really felt like I'd failed . . . He's also very keen on his own things – football, fishing, they don't involve me and he wouldn't give any of that up to help me . . . He doesn't really bother; takes life as it comes. He were getting fed up of me going on about it. His attitude is 'what's going to be's going to be'. I said 'you don't understand, you've got one already, it's alright for you'. When I was at me mum's [earlier temporary separation] he got in touch, said a welfare officer had helped him understand; but he didn't really. I don't think he really tried. I think if we'd had a child, we'd still be together. I can't imagine it though. I can't say really. I think maybe things would have been different . . . Stuart says one of the problems was me not accepting Jackie; feels I held that against him. Yes, I think that's true, I couldn't accept her as a daughter, but perhaps as a friend. I still find it difficult; he's got one and I haven't. It's awful to feel that but I do.

The fourth couple, Mr and Mrs Carter, separated quite early in the study; only the first interview was a joint one. At first follow-up Mrs Carter promised to be present although warning me on the telephone that things were difficult between them. She did not return for the interview, and despite many telephone contacts over the succeeding three years in which she promised to make an appointment, or get in touch with me 'a bit later on', she never kept these promises. I therefore received only the views of Mr Carter who saw me as agreed, and gave me details of their attendance for marriage guidance. The Carters were teachers; articulate and intelligent. When marital problems were mentioned at the Clinic a referral was made to a local psychologist. After several sessions the psychologist reported that in his view the marriage had no future, and he would help them to separate if that was what they wished. They did not, and did not return. Mrs Carter continued with investigations and treatment for her gynaecological problems long after their final separation.

Mr Carter spoke of their problems in the following way at the six-monthly interview, prior to the referral for marital help.

> At present I think she just wants to turn her back on the fertility problem . . . I still hope she'll come to terms with them. I don't think

she'll be going on with the Infertility Clinic . . . I don't think it's the investigations that've disturbed the marriage, but it's a crisis, sort of, that's made her rethink her role and expectations of life. She had this cosy progression from daughter to full-time student to wife without a break; it was broken by her failure to produce children, and, not having created a career, and being otherwise very tied to the home. She did say how fed up she got of being in the house so much.

It was clear that Mr Carter did indeed have fairly conventional expectations of his wife's role. He seemed to share the notion of their problems being, in large part at least, 'her failure'. The notion of crisis appeared apposite in this case. The failure of fertility led Mrs Carter, on Mr Carter's account, to a fairly wide-ranging reappraisal of her lifestyle: she took up employment for the first time, and began to pursue interests, including a new church, of her own choosing. Active sports, foreign holidays and, indeed, the role of working wife, all seemed to be at odds with his expectations. For Mrs Carter it seemed that questions of fertility were bound up with other important notions and self-images; the frustration of one leading to fundamental reviews of the others.

This was Mr Carter's perception of their situation on the last occasion we met.

Both came away [from the marital clinic] feeling the system was so incompetent, it gave us our first sense of comradeship for a while; but the feeling did not last and it was the last time we went . . . She often said 'you don't understand'. Infertility did make our relationship more difficult, particularly after she rebuffed any physical contact; so that is some exacerbation. When she felt footloose and doing things she would have done if single, infertility not a big factor; except as 'I might as well do other things instead'. It was fairly obvious; suddenly taking advantage of the freedom, filling the gap left by finding she could not start a family. That made the relationship go down hill quickly . . . [Infertility] just made everything else more difficult. By the breaking up, it wasn't an issue on the surface. It must still have been there, but it wasn't evident.

In their different ways the situations of the Carters and Traffords spoke eloquently of the extent to which fertility cannot be considered separately from key issues of gender role and the associated pronatalism discussed in Chapter 3. Childlessness in these cases provoked powerful feelings about expected roles; although Mrs Trafford had hardly begun to formulate them. Involuntary childlessness may test a marriage severely, not simply for the frustration of the desire to parent, but because of the impact it has on the partners' perceptions of what they expect from the marriage, and what might, in fact, be on offer.

All couples were specifically asked about their arguments. The phrasing of this question was deliberately in the classic mode of 'have you stopped beating your wife?'. It was hoped that this might be seen to be giving the couples permission to admit to having rows. Sixteen (53 per cent) of the men and 17 (57 per cent) of the women claimed to have noticed no difference in the frequency of their disagreements. Eight (27 per cent) of the men and seven (23 per cent) of their wives felt they disagreed less often than before deciding that they had a fertility problem.

> When we were going through it the slightest thing could upset the wife. If you really care you can't argue back as you'd do normally. You've got to be careful over everything you say.   (Mr Newsome)

However, the same perspective led another man to point out that they now rowed more than at that time.

> Rows were less frequent then; more sympathetic then because of that hanging over us. Just afraid of hurting each other more.
>
>   (Mr Coleman)

Similarly, several of those who had become parents mentioned that they now had more rows, which were related to their children, e.g. issues of discipline or of the husband taking a full share of responsibility.

Apart from the four couples mentioned earlier, all of the other childless couples claimed to row no more than before, or in some cases less.

> Haven't had a good row for a bit; we've got used to each other – quite an idyllic relationship now.   (Mr Lamb)

No universal effect of childlessness on disagreements between the partners emerged. For some it served as a major source of anxiety triggering bad feeling between husband and wife, in other cases it acted to discourage rows because of a heightened sense of mutual responsibility.

SEX AND CHILDLESSNESS

The impact of childlessness and its investigation on the sexual relationship is given substantial attention in the literature reviewed in Chapter 2. A majority of men (18, 60 per cent) and women (17, 57 per cent) interviewed felt that their sex lives had been adversely affected in some way. The other couples said that they had been unaffected. For all of the couples who reported an adverse effect, the critical time was during the investigations, rather than the whole period of infertility. The majority of those who reported a sexual relationship which remained the same over the period were still childless. Those who had since had a child appeared more ready to discuss this and report unsatisfactory experiences. The matter was not pursued if the couple chose only to respond in a minimal fashion in view of the already considerable personal exposure demanded by the interview. No positive effects were reported by the couples.

The most significant and frequently reported ill effect was the disappearance of spontaneity caused by the monitoring of intercourse required as part of the investigation. All the women, from the beginning of investigation, whether or not there was any reason for believing that their fertility might be impaired, were asked to keep a temperature chart on which was recorded the days on which periods came and on which there was sexual intercourse.

> Very anxious then; I remember thinking when doing the chart, 'is this normal? should we put some more in or scrub some out?' . . . Used to watch for the temperature change then have sex. That was terrible!
>
> (Mrs Truswell)

This loss of privacy seemed to affect some of the women; it was another way in which they were led to question their normality. Perhaps not surprisingly, the Grindrods, who came to the Clinic admitting a very unsatisfactory and infrequent sexual relationship, remarked that sex became not just dirty but pointless for Mrs Grindrod. This problem was not addressed by the Clinic, although admittedly it appeared to have no direct bearing on their infertility.

Sex was often described as becoming highly instrumental; it lost meaning as an expression of love or simple pleasure and became part of the treatment designed to produce a baby.

> It was very much that sex was purely for a family. It took the love and spontaneity out of it. These are the days we mustn't miss. It was every night for a week, then not again for a month. The longer it went on the worse it got. (Mr Mitchell)

> To a set time. It was all clinical and thermometers. It was pressure . . . You were afraid they were going to say 'you're not giving it a chance'.
>
> (Mrs Mitchell)

> As soon as you started making love, it was in your mind; 'is this the time we'll make a baby?' There were times I didn't feel like it, but I made myself. (Mrs Neal)

> Sex by numbers, that went on for a while. I got the feeling you were just a baby-making machine. When someone tells you 'this is the day'.
>
> (Mr Crow)

Most of the couples described the effects as only temporary, resolved when the BBT in particular was discontinued. But for one couple at least there were longer term results, even after the arrival of a baby.

> Definitely it did! Beforehand it suffered; previously we had it twice in six months, now it's down to once a year. It's never been the same, but it'll come back. [*He laughed and went out to make tea.*]
>
> (Mr Newsome)

> Before it was good, but it really became terrible. Prior to problems it was fine, seriously it was fine, hasn't ever been the same. Can't get back to where it was before. It does worry me at times. Eventually I gave up taking my temperature it got so terrrible. What's the point in making love if you can't have a baby? We were just doing it for a baby, not getting any satisfaction. It's funny you asking that!   (Mrs Newsome)

Substantial ill-feeling was generated amongst some of the couples who kept the charts carefully, only to find that the Clinic doctor paid them scant regard. It was widely felt that the cost to the couple was either unrecognised or ignored. If anxiety does indeed prejudice fertility, the insistence on the keeping of a temperature chart by the wife, often for very long periods of time, seems possibly counterproductive. In order to minimise the stress experienced by the couple under investigation, and possibly thus enhance their chances of conception, an infertility clinic might be well advised to use this particular investigation much more selectively, and for shorter periods, than currently is often the case. Where uncertain ovulation is being investigated the temperature chart might be required for an extended period. In this case, medical staff might suggest that the woman no longer records intercourse, once it has been established that the couple are able to time intercourse appropriately. This is an instance in which routinised medical practice might, with advantage, become more individualised.

This Clinic did not, however, routinely use the post-coital test at the time of this investigation. This, as described elsewhere (Appendix III), requires a couple to have intercourse within a prescribed period of hours prior to attending the Clinic when a sample of cervical mucus is taken from the woman to assess semen compatibility and sperm adequacy. Some practices described in the literature seem particularly insensitive; e.g. Philipp and Carruthers (1981) require that couples attending their clinic have intercourse the night before the first appointment and come prepared for the PCT as one of the initial tests; Menning (1977) reports that clinics in the United States sometimes expect intercourse to be performed in the clinic to ensure the earliest possible PCT. The demands made in this Clinic were not therefore as great as others reported in the literature.

Despite the emphasis given to sex in books concerning the management of infertility, it appeared from this study that the complaints found in 'consumer' accounts discussed elsewhere are not unique. Whatever the textbook importance of a physically and emotionally adequate sex life for those with a fertility problem, consideration of these matters did not figure greatly in the considerations of this Clinic, although they caused the couples considerable concern.

CHILDLESSNESS AND OTHER RELATIONSHIPS

In the preceding sections the focus has been on the individual and the couple, but it has been necessary to comment on the effect of the attitudes and expectations of other people to the couple's childlessness. In this section specific attention will be paid to ways in which childlessness seemed to affect other relationships of importance to the couples involved.

The extent to which couples felt that their infertility affected, and was affected by, other people was, to a very great extent, determined by the numbers and closeness of the people whom they took into their confidence. As already discussed, there was substantial variation in the readiness with which they confided in this way.

Parents

For many couples a principal source of pressure to have children came, they felt, from their parents (see also Chapter 5). Erikson (1950) emphasises the importance of 'generativity' in transition to full adult status, by which he means the experience of parenting.

Mahlstedt (1985) notes the impact of losing a 'stake in the future', as it is popularly described. These drives do not attain their full satisfaction with parenthood, it seems. There is the next, and possibly equally urgent, need to see one's own children having children.

At the second interview, seven couples mentioned that the husband's parents were upset at their childlessness, and seven mentioned the wife's parents. At this stage both sets of parents had not been told of the problems in all cases. In two cases in which parents were alive, the men never confided in their parents at all. At the final interview, five couples said that their parents had been adversely affected in some way; upset, worried, afraid of never having a grandchild.

> I feel under a lot of pressure from the in-laws. His brother had a boy and a girl in the time we've been trying. My parents are very upset . . . I still feel Dick's parents think I brought it on myself; 'we've got grand-

children, why does she want to bother?' They're not really sympathetic. Do you know, his mother dragged me round toy shops at Christmas, and never thought it might upset me, not having children? . . . I felt pressured by Dick's parents . . . they made me feel inadequate; I'd never be anything to them until I had a child . . . I think I got quite paranoid about them at one time.   (Mrs Mitchell)

These feelings were more vehemently expressed than in most cases, but were not atypical of the pressures experienced. As in other respects, the impression given was that wives felt these pressures more keenly than their husbands. Most made the point that it was not just a matter that women were more sensitive to the hints or enquiries, but that these things were in fact much more likely to be directed towards them. The Butlers noted this difference.

I never felt under much pressure.   (Mr Butler)

I felt the pressure, particularly from your parents. She [mother-in-law] arranged the acupuncturist, and she's on the lookout for herbal remedies, anything.   (Mrs Butler)

Some couples clearly saw their parents as a factor in their environment to be controlled in order to manage their own emotional pressures.

The parents put a lot of pressure on – we never told my mum.
                                                                       (Mr Diamond)

It upset my mum, but she's about the only one we told.
                                                                     (Mrs Diamond)

The parents want grandchildren, but we don't want to go into it all the time. It all adds to the pressure. Parents just don't know.   (Mr Crow)

It would be wrong to give the impression that all parents were seen as figures increasing the emotional pressure felt by the couples. Most claimed that their parents were very sympathetic towards their plight (see Chapter 5). In several cases a distinction was drawn which clarifies this apparent inconsistency. Parents were sometimes seen as very concerned and upset for their children, but this felt like an increase in the emotional pressure experienced by the childless couple, rather than a sharing of the burden.

They're upset, very upset . . . traumatic having to tell them; all crying an' that.   (Mr Green)

Mel's parents are concerned; they try to reassure us; they probably think we're too tense, and the solution will come through relaxing more!
                                                                      (Mrs Monk)

The smallest group of responses was those which unequivocally spoke of the positive role of the parents in supporting them.

> Affected my family – we're very close to them . . . talk a lot about it. Mother's very keen for us to succeed . . . her mind's been put at rest through coming to the Clinic. She couldn't see why her daughter shouldn't have as easy a time as she had. I'm pleased that I can discuss it with her.   (Mrs Ivy)

> My parents have no grandchildren . . . We both get on well with our own parents as well as the in-laws; very close family. We discuss it all easily, very involved, share the problem and report to them on appointments; they want to know all about it.   (Mr Ivy)

The general impression given was that the wife's mother was an important figure in this context, but perhaps less central and less likely to be invariably supportive than other studies have painted her (e.g. Young and Wilmott 1957, 1973, Voysey 1975, Oakley 1979, Pahl 1984). The ambivalence raised by this very personal area of a marriage, and the efforts frequently made by the wife to protect her husband from the 'stigma' of sterility, might be important factors. The distance which crept in between some of the wives and their mothers may have been an important contributory element in the trauma of childlessness.

Family and friends

Strong feelings were also raised by relationships with other members of the family and personal friends, which, as with parents, were not always helpful and supportive, regardless of the generally positive assessment of their attitudes.

The couples were asked to try to put themselves in the position of others who knew them well, and picture how these others would describe them, as another perspective on the effects of infertility. Naturally, as several couples observed, they would not be friends unless they had fairly positive views. However, some of the couples took the opportunity to make some interesting comments on how their experiences might have affected them in the eyes of others, as well as the attitudes they encountered as childless couples.

As already indicated, the couples felt that, on the whole, other people had been fairly sympathetic. In discussion, less positive attitudes were mentioned. Only a minority of the couples volunteered that they had received active sympathy and concern for their plight.

> I think they felt sorry for us. We're god-parents to lots of kids. I think

they all sympathised with us . . . were just asking questions, not going too deep. A lot of people are afraid to ask.   (Mr David)

Close friends were a bit wary; afraid of upsetting Cathy; felt like being an intruder to them I think.   (Mr Mitchell)

Typically, these quotations show the extent to which this concern was so often felt to be tinged with reticence. Reluctance to talk about childlessness created substantial barriers for most of these couples, increasing their sense of isolation.

Previously [to having child] people were thoughtless. They don't know what to say. Only people in the same position can talk about it . . . the majority are kind but the odd loud mouth ridicules you.   (Mr Quick)

It was recognised that this isolation was, at least in part, self-imposed, although no less keenly felt for that.

It seems to be pushed; soon as it involves you it hits you, and people seem to be asking suddenly. Not told anyone, not even her parents . . . some friends ask, but not told them the results . . . only told one cousin. We're afraid of people joking about it. You can't expect much sympathy.   (Mr Urmston)

Didn't discuss it with them [friends] very much, kept it to ourselves. Because if other people know they tend to keep on about it. It's difficult enough without lots of people asking.   (Mrs Menzies)

The isolation itself caused difficulties in getting events associated with infertility in perspective. The Newsomes put this point well on the first follow-up visit.

Other people's attitudes hurt.   (Mr Newsome)

I don't want people asking; I'd rather come out with it myself, and not be asked.   (Mrs Newsome)

Problem is not so much the doctors and nurses, it's them out there, Joe Public; you don't think about it until it happens.   (Mr Newsome)

I think there should be somewhere you can go to talk to someone about it, who's been through it. An association for it. It's not something you talk to everyone about. It's not a nice thing to admit. No one knows as much as we've told you. . . Don't talk to a lot of people. Keep on talking like this, and when you've gone it will be OK. [*i.e. the sex problem they had discussed.*]   (Mrs Newsome)

There was a feeling that others were not simply being insensitive, but that pronatalist attitudes were so strong that non-parents were seen as inferior in a generalised way; the 'freemasonry of the fertile' of which Robinson (1982) writes.

> I hated being lectured to by people with kids. People get on their high horses talking about kids. (Mr Keith)

> People can be very insensitive. Everyone with children assumes everyone can have children if they want them. (Mr Crow)

> A lot of it is you're expected to have them. Anyone who doesn't is seen to be abnormal. (Mrs Crow)

One aspect of this 'freemasonry' is the practical one of sharing such a major 'interest' in common.

> It got to be a strain. With a baby you have a reason to go and see someone. (Mrs Newsome)

> We've lots of friends; kept us going . . . it's maybe easier now as all the friends have children too. We're the same now. (Mr Carver)

> Not many friends – they're mostly young families or old round here. Don't go out with people locally; not many our age. (Mrs Kitchen)

Only one couple, the Neals, expressed an awareness of these pressures in terms of expectations of conventional sex-linked roles. (The Neals were a working-class couple; he was a miner and she was a cleaner, certainly not middle-class 'trendies'.)

> I've quietly settled down into family life. See a lot more of the family, and take more interest in my brothers' and sisters' families. They bring their kids down now which they never did before. (Mr Neal)

> We seem to have arrived! Before they never came round. A lot of them think I should put up with this 'woman's role' thing like they do. They want nothing but being a mum. I'm not a second class citizen; there's a lot more I'd like to do. But having said that, I'll miss her when she goes to school. (Mrs Neal)

Mrs Butler also spoke strongly of her irritation with those who, in her view, saw her returning to work soon after her daughter's birth and employing a nanny as particularly blameworthy in one who had found difficulty in having a child at all.

In some cases the longer-term effects appeared to include having less contact with friends, partly through the drawing away that had occurred at the time of the infertility investigation, even when, as in the two cases quoted below, they subsequently had children.

> They think we're lucky materially . . . not got deep friendships; we're not first on the list for rave-ups.   (Mr Mitchell)

> Only see the family now. I kept away from friends, it hurt so much.
>   (Mrs Newsome)

Fortunately, none of the women had the same experience as was recounted at a NAC meeting. This lady described how one of her closest 'friends', a neighbour who had started to try for a child herself, came up to her one day and said, 'I don't think I should have anything to do with people like you, now I'm wanting a baby.' The involuntarily childless woman concerned described feeling just as if she was carrying some contagious disease. This was the most striking illustration of some of the extraordinarily primitive attitudes that lie close to the surface of childbirth, which could trigger some very difficult interactions during the time of childlessness.

Domestic pets

The issue of pets may be seen as sensitive by some childless people. For several years the National Association for the Childless ran a column in its magazine *NACK* concerning members' pets. The idea was not uncontroversial and has since been dropped. To judge from the regularity and size of the column, however, as well as the correspondence, it enjoyed a substantial following amongst readers.

The Butlers, although they owned a dog whilst still childless, mentioned having affection for animals as child substitutes as part of their stereotype of the 'Childless Couple' – a view which, I suspect, is widely held. Anecdotal evidence suggests that pet ownership does meet certain needs to parent. This appears to be equally as true for some people who are parents as for some who are not. Like the evidence regarding the occurrence of conception after adoption, this common stereotype might have as much to do with the visibility of an already stigmatised group as any real differences.

Baum (1980), however, noted that amongst her voluntarily childless couples pet ownership was 73 per cent above average. Young and Wilmott (1973) found that 58 per cent of their 1,900 couples in the South East owned one or more pets, of whom 25 per cent owned dogs. In this study, 18 (60 per cent) are pet owners; not a surprisingly large proportion, although 40 per cent owned one or more dogs, the animal perhaps best suited to the role of child substitute. There were two couples for whom there was striking evidence that pets might play an important role of this kind for some childless people. The Grindrods, who remained childless, described their miniature Shetland sheep dog as 'ruined – he's our baby!'. The Menzies at the first interview had on display Father's Day cards to Mr Menzies 'from' the dog. At the second interview it was the dog's birthday; it had received five carefully chosen and displayed cards. This attachment seemed not to be diminished or made less sentimental by their having a child. Twelve (40 per cent) of the couples, however, had no pets at all.

There was no strong evidence that these childless couples were using pets to an unusual extent as child substitutes.

SUMMARY

The evidence presented in this chapter confirms the substantial impact of the experience of childlessness. This impact is not only felt individually, but also in the marriage and other relationships.

These emotional reactions and experiences are not substantially different to those presented in Chapter 5. The concern was to demonstrate the persistence of these feelings, the changes that took place over time, and the way in which the experience of investigation compounded them in certain respects.

It cannot be said that all individuals feel the impact in the same way or to the same extent; few are immune, however, from the personal distress described here. The difference between the way in which it appears to affect men and women was marked. Women were more likely to report personal anguish, depression, isolation and jealousy. Husbands more often spoke of distress at a diagnosis of subfertility on their part, the distress caused to their wives or their anger at perceived deficiencies in the service provided in the Clinic. Whilst the men appeared to become less distressed over time, whatever the investigations produced, only those women who became pregnant became less distressed. For men, apparently, time healed more quickly. Childlessness also appeared, for men and women, to affect adversely their ability to cope adequately, in their own eyes, with normal social relationships and obligations. Women were especially likely to report feeling depressed and isolated as a result of their childlessness. A diagnosis of infertility appeared to threaten the man's sexual identity more fundamentally. The woman was more likely to express her feelings in terms of personal distress or failing in an obligation to the husband. None of the infertile men expressed a sense of failing his wife. Overall, a strong impression was given that the experience of infertility is a very different one for men and women. Internalised and external expectations appear to combine in 'protecting' the man more than his wife in an infertile marriage.

The concepts of bereavement are useful in understanding the experience of childlessness over its natural course. However, the process is best understood in terms of common and significant reactions, not as a predetermined succession of stages.

The marriages were put under substantial strain both by the experience of childlessness and its treatment. On balance, the evidence suggested that this was a crisis, the effects of which were to undermine already weak relationships and to strengthen those that were already sound and supportive. There was little to suggest that childlessness might be expected on its own to be a major cause of marital breakdown. There was a marked, adverse effect on the sexual relationship of childless couples, which seemed to relate particularly to the process of investigation, rather than the childlessness *per se*.

Other relationships were also affected by a couple's childlessness. The personal nature of the experience often made it very difficult for couples to seek help and support in the places they would normally have looked. Parents in particular were likely to have their own investment in their children's fertility, which called their ability to provide support into question. The position of siblings with children might be an added source of pressure. Even relationships with friends might become difficult, partly because of the pervasiveness of social attitudes towards fertility and parenthood. The experience of childlessness struck at the heart of many issues and social relationships of fundamental importance to these couples; in the light of this, understanding the distress and confusion that so often appeared is not difficult.

This distress and confusion cannot be confidently attached exclusively to the childlessness or the investigation and treatment that the couples underwent at the Infertility Clinic. The separation of the elements of this experience must be artificial. The succeeding chapter will present their views of the process as it seemed to them, both at the time and subsequently, and the changes in these views which appeared to take place as time passed and situations changed. Whilst this will enable some comments to be made on aspects of the process which appear to exacerbate the distress of childlessness, the possibility remains that many of the concerns were epiphenomenal, mere representations of the distress.

7 Undergoing childlessness

In a study of this sort it is not possible to isolate the effects of childlessness which concern fertility status and those which are directly related to the process of investigation. Both are part of the reality with which the couples are working and trying to cope successfully. This chapter will present their experiences of being investigated and treated for childlessness in this Infertility Clinic, as it operated at the time of the study, which is now much changed.

Over a period of three years or more it is to be expected that the views of the couples should change in some ways. Their feelings are presented as expressed to me, for the perspective it gives of those undergoing sophisticated medical procedures in the emotional climate described in the previous chapter. Only if these feelings are understood and acknowledged can a properly sensitive service be offered.

There were changes in the way that individuals viewed the services they received. Using the model of bereavement again is helpful in putting the initial level of dissatisfaction in a context of early anger and protest at the situation which necessitated such procedures. One illustration of this is that the number of complaints about the service provided by the Clinic diminished with the passing of time; however, the number of positive things the couples had to say about their treatment also diminished. This was not, therefore, an indication of recollection becoming simply 'rose tinted'; rather the Clinic assumed a lesser importance in their eyes as test results, positive or negative, were obtained. There was little to suggest that the extent of criticism was related to the success, or otherwise, of treatment. Some of the fiercest critics of the Clinic became parents, just as some of the staunchest supporters failed to have children.

The satisfaction of these couples with their experience of the Clinic will be discussed in some detail. Couples will not be classified as 'satisfied' or 'dissatisfied', however: such an approach is too simplistic to represent adequately the complexities of their experience, let alone the complex interactions involved in patients negotiating their relationships with a hospital system (see Mauksch 1972 and Stimson and Webb 1975 for general discussions of these issues). Their experiences will be presented in their richness and variety, and their inconsistency in some cases. The concern is to clarify those components of the process which couples experienced as helpful and those which were experienced as unhelpful.

UNDERSTANDING AND CO-OPERATION

Substantial concerns arose over the way in which Clinic staff conveyed information concerning the couples' test results. These concerns are not surprising both in view of the technical nature of the information being considered and in view of consistent findings in other fields that patients frequently complain of not having medical information explained to them in comprehensible terms. Cartwright and Anderson (1981) found a quarter of GPs' patients dissatisfied with the way their doctors explained their medical condition when consulted. Eisenthal and Lazare (1976), Thomas (1978), Putnam *et al.* (1979) and Treadway (1983) provide examples of studies in general practice, psychiatric clinic, and hospital out-patients, all of which confirm that patients will be more satisfied in their encounters with doctors when they feel they understand and have been understood.

What doctors do is less important than how they interact.
(Yourti *et al.* 1976)

At both first and second follow-up interviews the couples were asked to explain their medical situation as a means of gauging their understanding. On the first of these occasions, 25 (83 per cent) explained their position accurately (although not necessarily having the precise words to explain the diagnosis), five (17 per cent) appeared only partly to understand the situation. This seemed to be a very good result in contrast to the experiences described in the studies mentioned previously. The partial understandings were those couples who appeared to have grasped some of the information but not all the important items. One of these was the couple whose situation was outlined in Chapter 5, in which Mr Mitchell denied his oligospermia diagnosis and they both denied their almost certain conception by DI. At this stage the Mitchells commented:

I'm normal at least. (Mr Mitchell)

He's not really a problem as such. (Mrs Mitchell)

Although they had yet to be given DI at this stage, the denial was apparently already mobilised to defend Mr Mitchell against any presumption of impaired masculinity. One may assume that the denial was intentional rather than unconscious on the basis of his undoubted intelligence, the rather less certain response of his wife, and the fact that he went along with the referral for DI treatment.

Mr Crow also gave an inaccurate impression of his fertility. He described his semen as '5-star rocket fuel', at a time when he had already been diagnosed as severely oligospermic. Subsequently he underwent hormonal treatment, but they did not consider DI. His wife had substantial problems also, which they pursued throughout the period of the study, mainly in private treatment at the associated University Clinic. Mr Crow was perhaps the most angry and critical of the people interviewed in the study. The denial could have been less conscious in this case. The impression given, however, was that his anger focused mainly on being found to be subfertile. Mr Crow was especially critical of what he perceived as an atmosphere in the Clinic which excluded men and ignored their feelings almost totally. Both of these cases, then, suggested that failure to understand was explicable in terms of the emotional consequences for the men of a diagnosis of subfertility, and not necessarily or simply in failures among staff.

In the other three cases in which the patients only partly understood the situation, the women concerned had multiple problems of tubal occlusion and ovulatory dysfunction, and seemed not to have grasped the complexity of the situation. One, an articulate, middle-class woman, Mrs Lamb, had quite clearly fastened on to one aspect of the explanation and wholly misapplied it. She spoke of 'odd bumps and irregularities', thinking these were structural problems of her internal organs when the main problem was an irregular menstrual cycle. It seemed that the phrase she used might have been the doctor's description of the temperature chart.

At this same stage the couples were asked to recount the investigations and treatments they had undergone and their answers compared with the medical notes. Only three of the men failed to provide an accurate account of their experiences. Two have already been discussed. The other had been for genetic counselling which was not clearly recalled and understood. Five of the women failed accurately to recall the tests and treatment administered. Some tests were apparently not recalled, despite prompting. Many could not name the actual tests or drugs but were able to describe their nature or purpose. One treatment that seemed to cause some confusion was the drug, Danazol, given for endometriosis. Three women who had received it seemed unsure of its purpose, and, perhaps of more concern, two of these seemed not to appreciate that the drug's action meant that conception was impossible whilst it was being taken.

The couples were asked at first follow-up if there were aspects of the process which they had felt unable to accept. The circumstances in which some couples withdrew from further treatment will be discussed later. The picture that emerged was one of full co-operation with the Clinic. None of the men indicated that they had not been able to co-operate fully. However, given the number of those who had very little contact with the Clinic this cannot be seen as an indication of whole-hearted general involvement; rather it suggests that there was no specific demand made of these men which prompted them into not co-operating. Whether the Clinic asked enough of them is an issue to be considered later.

Three of the women said that they had not felt able to continue with the temperature charting for as long as the Clinic expected. This issue has been mentioned above (p. 134). Each felt that this procedure increased the stress of infertility for them, and the results were not used enough by the doctors to make it worth while.

When couples were asked directly if there had been anything they had not understood, a less positive picture emerged. Half of the men and 16 (55 per cent) of the women felt that there were things that they had not understood about the procedures. Four of the men (in addition to the two men discussed above) mentioned technicalities of the semen analysis result as not clear. Four said they did not understand the purpose of the testicular biopsy, and two more the results of that biopsy. Amongst the women four mentioned specific results as not being clear, and two the purpose of some of the procedures.

Three couples commented that one of the strengths of the Clinic was its willingness to explain what is happening so that patients can understand. This did not, however, seem to be the general experience. Altogether, 12 (40 per cent) complained of a general sense of not knowing what was happening to them or why. One woman, Mrs Green, put this feeling succinctly, laying the blame firmly on the Clinic staff:

They don't explain; they think we're too thick to understand.

The Colemans put the same feeling thus:

We had to ask for answers; never explained until we asked.

(Mr Coleman)

They wouldn't even explain the reason for the delay in getting the results of the tests. We only really knew what was going on as a result of reading a book . . . Saw one doctor most of the time; we couldn't understand her and she couldn't understand us. She couldn't understand others' feelings at all. (Mrs Coleman)

I have chosen to quote the feelings of this couple although they did emphasise the role of a doctor whom they felt to have been particularly unhelpful. There was no evidence of a 'doctor-specific' effect in relation to complaints of this category.

It was striking that at second follow-up this was one of the concerns that appeared to diminish with distance. Only one couple at this stage complained about this feature of their treatment.

There were also three couples who specifically mentioned that the Clinic staff did explain things adequately in their experience.

> Last time we went [doctor] explained DI clearly; no trying to make you feel better, no soft soaping; better than being led on.   (Mr Monk)

> Good in explaining, telling you about the results and what was wrong.
>
> (Mrs Monk)

The commitment of the couples could be gauged in some degree from the limits they put, after six months had passed, on their attendance at the Clinic. Only seven (27 per cent) of the couples had a limit in mind. The shortest period mentioned was a further year, the longest was four years. Five of these periods were selected on the basis of the age of the wife and concerns about safe child-bearing and adoption limits. For all the frustration at the slow pace at which investigation proceeded, there was little evidence that this frustration led to reduced commitment.

Similarly, any perceived failings in transmitting clear information about the progress of investigation, did not reduce commitment to the procedure. These couples were, in some cases, willing to pay a substantial price in pursuit of their goal.

EXPECTATIONS AND EXPERIENCE

None had previously been investigated for infertility – one of the criteria for selection. It is not, then, surprising that a substantial proportion felt unprepared for what becoming a patient at the Clinic would involve. Fourteen (47 per cent) of the men felt unprepared and 15 (50 per cent) of the women; 9 (30 per cent) of the men felt that the Clinic was not what they expected and 13 (43 per cent) of the women.

In looking at the extent to which the service satisfied their hopes and expectations, it might be useful to summarise the positive and negative things the couples had to say, and the frequency with which these observations were made in interviews. In order to facilitate comprehensive responses at each stage, a number of questions were asked. The responses to these have been combined as positive and negative feelings, 'compliments' and 'complaints'. This approach was designed to reduce the halo effect whereby it might be expected that those who were successful in having a child, if simply asked for an opinion of the Clinic, might be blandly uncritical, and possibly those who were unsuccessful the reverse.

Only a small minority could be fairly categorised overall as 'satisfied' or 'dissatisfied'. For the majority the picture was one with good and bad patches in its design. The focus for analysis will be on clarifying elements in the process which met with more or less approval, and which possibly helped or hindered the full participation of the patients in their treatment.

As may be seen from Tables 7.1 and 7.2, complaints at both stages of interviewing outnumbered compliments almost two-fold. (This is not to suggest that the items can in any sense be regarded as of equal weight.) Several factors might lead to this result.

Firstly, the infertility service at the start of the study was an 'unofficial' clinic, in the National Health Service sense that it ran at the instigation of the consultant and was staffed out of the goodwill of various professionals, some employed by the hospital and others by the university, but without formal recognition as part of the funded activity of the hospital. This inevitably exacerbated problems of underfunding and inadequate staffing in the NHS. This improved later when the Clinic gained formal status, which enabled it to move from the ante-natal clinic, which had provoked substantial criticism, to the gynaecology department of the hospital. On the

Table 7.1 Compliments

	FU1		FU2	
	N=30	%	N=28	%
Staff attitudes	15	50	10	36
Treatment/progress	15	50	4	14
Results/hope	10	33	3	11
Explanation/information	6	21	6	21
Professional/thorough	5	18	6	21
Others[1]	3	10	3	11
Totals	54		32	
Nil[2]	4	13	8	29

N.B. Multiple replies give totals in excess of 100 per cent.

1. FU1:   Speed of investigation (3).
    FU2:   Speed of investigation (2), seeing monitor during HSG (1).
2. 'Nil': No good things to say, and the only reply given.

Table 7.2 Complaints

	FU1		FU2	
	N=30	%	N=28	%
Explanation/information	17	57	5	18
Waiting time	16	53	7	25
Duration of process	16	53	13	46
Changing doctors	7	23	5	18
Administration	7	23	8	29
Staff attitudes	7	23	5	18
Husband left out	6	20	6	20
Difficult investigation	5	17	4	14
Consultant not seen	4	14	3	11
Abortions	2	7	3	11
Others[1]	11	37	6	21
Totals	98		65	
Nil[2]	5	17	4	14

N.B. Multiple replies give totals in excess of 100 per cent.

1. FU1: Short consultations (2), lack of privacy (3), setting (2), ignoring feelings (2), poor GP contact (1), uncomfortable waiting room (1).
   FU2: Setting (2), travelling (2), visiting (1), lack of privacy (1).
2. 'Nil': No critical things to say, and the only reply given.

staffing side, ante-natal nursing staff with their focus on babies could be replaced with gynaecology nurses. The Senior House Officer (SHO) in pathology has usually been replaced with a gynaecological SHO, and often with other research staff at a more senior level. The medical staffing improvements have been via university and research, not National Health Service, funds. Organisationally, the service was sharpened, and the basic investigations were completed in two appointments in most cases, although laparoscopy still involved long waiting lists. These changes were commended by several couples who experienced them, although they are not reflected in the results as they affected only a few couples at a very late stage.

Secondly, it is perhaps to be expected that, when asked to air their opinions, particularly in relation to a preoccupying and anxiety-laden condition such as infertility, it will be the negatives that come first to mind. They perhaps assume the character of a vehicle for many of the bad feelings associated with the childlessness itself. It should be said, in comparison, that a recent opinion poll survey of hospital in- and out-patients found that 88 per cent were fairly/very satisfied; a better result than this study obtained (NAHA 1987).

Thirdly, medical encounters being charged with disparities of power are likely to attract hostility, especially from those whose condition is peculiarly powerless. This may be taken to apply to the gender axis also. The distinction between the sexes is not always made in this discussion as comments were made in joint interviews, and whilst the man or woman answered it was often clear that he or she spoke for the partner as well. The extent of agreement was not tested formally; the views are therefore presented as those of individuals whilst attributing the incidence of these views to couples. If anything, the men were more forceful in presenting their discontent, despite (and in a few cases, because of) their lesser involvement.

Fourthly, as Cartwright and Anderson (1981) observe, there is a wide-spread and increasing tendency in our post-Nader society not to accept uncomplainingly the ministrations of professionals. They noted a sub-stantial increase in the readiness of patients to complain about their GPs in the 13 years separating their two studies, conducted in 1964 and 1977. Given the way in which these couples were selected (see Chapter 4) there is no reason to believe that the discontented were unduly represented in this study.

The second general feature which is immediately apparent from Tables 7.1 and 7.2 is that both complaints and compliments became less frequent over time. The analogy with bereavement is relevant in understanding this phenomenon. Early reactions to loss, according to Murray Parkes (1986), notably include protest and anger. It might be expected, therefore, that initial comments would be particularly unfavourable to the Clinic; hence the value of obtaining views at greater remove from the experience. The complaints seemed, however, to diminish less than the positive comments. Whilst the number of those who said they only had positive feelings when asked if they had any criticisms about the Clinic service stayed constant over the period, the number of those couples who had only negative feelings almost doubled to one-third.

Naturally, the parents in the sample at the final interview, preoccupied with the pressures of parenthood and having achieved the object of attending the Clinic, would have every reason to put the bad experiences behind them. But it was not the case that the parents now felt positively, and the childless negatively, towards the Clinic. Ardent champions were to be found amongst the childless as well as fierce critics amongst the parents. Of the nine who could offer no positive comments on the service at final interview, four had become parents. However, it is the case that the majority (77 per cent) of positive comments made at final interview came from the parents. Of the adverse comments, 65 per cent were recorded by parents. In both areas the childless were less likely to comment about the Clinic.

Although there can be no sensible measure of the relative importance of one criticism over another, whilst some of the criticisms were made by only a few of the respondents, this should not be taken to diminish the importance of the feeling. For example, although only a minority had distressing experiences in connection with abortion, the force of their feelings might be said to deserve as much attention as the greater number who complained about lack of information. In that sense it could be said to be of at least equal 'importance' to the reputation and standing of the infertility service.

In presenting views, positive comments will be given first. No further attempt will be made to quantify either positive or negative feelings. It should also be remembered that this study did not set out to evaluate a particular clinical service (which, in any event, has changed substantially since the time of the study) but rather to elucidate the positive and negative factors in the childless couples' experience, which are likely to be replicated at other hospital services. The comments to be discussed do not, therefore, seek to isolate the impact of specific members of staff or parts of this service. Even in such a small group recruited over a fairly short time span, there were substantial variations in the particulars of their circumstances, investigation and treatment which would invalidate any such aim.

Staff attitudes

It was noticeable that this was one of the most positive features of the Clinic mentioned at the second interview. By the last interview this still accounted for almost one-third of all the positive comments. The number of couples who singled out this feature for praise fell, as with all the compliments. It is not being suggested that the couples necessarily felt less positively, simply that the experience seemed to recede in 'visibility'.

> It's been very good, they've put you at ease. The doctors were very nice.
> (Mrs Menzies)

> The place is nice; the nurses an' that. (Mrs David)

> [It] has to be one of the friendliest hospitals. [The consultant] couldn't do any more to help, himself. (Mrs Underwood)

Most of the positive comments were made by the wives.

For adverse comment, the level remained constant. The most frequent complaint regarding staff attitudes was the feeling some patients reported of being patronised.

> Got very angry with the doctor's attitude; felt belittled by him.
>
> (Mr Young)

A particularly bad encounter was certain to taint the whole experience, as happened with the Newsomes, who did have a child.

> On assessment day the sister shouts across the Clinic 'Are you the infertility lady?' She treated me like a kid. Some of the nurses are very patronising in their attitudes.   (Mrs Newsome)

In one case there arose the issue of what might be expected of the patient to be considered 'suitable' for infertility treatment.

> Manny's deaf and dumb; been like it since he was born. I didn't say anything about it at the hospital. I thought he [doctor] was already shocked at me wanting children and not being married an' that; if I'd come out and said 'he's disabled' as well, well I thought that'd be it.
>
> (Mrs Holt)

Their not being married was subsequently used, along with the severity of her problems and her age (not, however, his disability), as a reason for removing her from the IVF programme waiting list. Although in a sense quite an extreme situation, this did point up the extent to which the Clinic appeared likely to discriminate against those without fairly conventional personal situations. As discussed in relation to the 'hidden childless' who do not seek specialist help, it might be that this expectation of conventional social attitudes is a powerful influence upon those who find their way to the Infertility Clinic. The removal of Mrs Holt from the IVF list was the only overt sign of such attitudes. It was clear that they were a strong expectation in Mrs Holt's mind.

Overall, considerably more of the couples felt that the staff were concerned and sympathetic than felt that they were not.

Professional approach

The comments on this aspect of the service remained fairly constant.

> You know you're getting the best treatment available, that all the necessary drugs and treatments are available and will be provided.
>
> (Mr Butler)

> What was done was done very professionally.   (Mr Truswell)

The confidence that the Clinic was up-to-date and knew all the current developments was important.

> You know it's one of the best places in the country: know there's nowhere better you can go.   (Mr David)

Only one couple decided to go privately to the attached University Clinic, and they were anxious to point out that this was to avoid the worst delays, not in the expectation that they would get better medical treatment.

> Felt at last someone was doing something about it. I'd been messed around for so long before that. Ever since my periods started, I saw lots of doctors who did nothing. I was trying to convince everyone there was something wrong. Once I got to the [Hospital] I knew somebody was looking at things. I felt they were doing something, and sooner or later they'd tell me 'you can' or 'you can't' – you'd know one way or the other.   (Mrs Neal)

None of the couples directly accused the Clinic of being unprofessional in their approach. Some of the harsher criticisms that are noted later could, however, almost be said to amount to such a charge.

Treatment/progress

This is, of course, the central criterion by which patients are likely to judge the quality of the service they receive. However, as has been noted, this was not just measured crudely by whether or not the couple were able to have a child. To that extent it was clear that the complexity of the problems many faced was appreciated, and there was no evidence of unrealistic expectations of what might be achieved. In the case of male infertility there seemed to be a general assumption that this would be untreatable. By the time of the last interview most of the couples had ceased treatment, as may be seen from Figure 4.1. It is not, therefore, surprising that satisfaction with specific treatments ceased to figure in their comments about the Clinic.

> Pleased with what's happening; hope the result is as pleasing. Still quite confident, perhaps a bit more as drugs are now a possibility.   (Mr Ivy)

It was noted several times that 'things were getting on at last'. One aspect of this feeling was the relief when no major problem was uncovered by the investigation.

> Just pleased that we've gone after putting it off for so long. We didn't want to face up to the truth; pleased that they've looked around and not found anything really serious.   (Mr Lamb)

Even where the result was not what might have been hoped, for some couples the result was preferable to the uncertainty. 'At least you know', as Mr Urmston put it, who was found to be oligospermic.

> I went to get peace of mind, knowing the position.   (Mrs Underwood)

> Knowing what's wrong was like a big weight off my shoulders.
>
> (Mrs Thurston)

> They were good really, but never gave us an answer. Not their fault, of course, but you feel, what do I mean? bitter . . . or angry maybe, if you don't really know. They said 'we can't say definitely you won't' but they made it clear it was very unlikely.   (Mr Green)

Results/hope

This category of comments was closely linked with the previous group. At the first interview it was often noted that going to the Clinic gave the couple some hope that they would eventually have a child.

> Gives us a little more hope.   (Mrs Monk)

Part of this hope was the clarification of the nature or scope of their problem, if any.

> Know a bit more where we stand now; the direction we're going in.
>
> (Mr Turner)

Even where the hope proved to be false, having made the attempt was important.

> It gave me a chance, that's it really.   (Mrs Trafford)

Where positive results were achieved that person, as expected, would declare his or her personal sense of relief.

> I enjoyed it all because it achieved something.   (Mrs Butler)

In general terms, the Clinic gave its patients hope and optimism, without seeming unrealistic. Although many criticisms were voiced, most couples felt that if they were to become parents they could do no better than attend this Clinic.

> We're probably in good hands. They're really good at [the Hospital]. We refused the offer of private treatment paid for by the in-laws; think they're as good as anyone, better than most.   (Mrs Lamb)

Explanation/information

The falling off of criticism of the Clinic's perceived failings in communicating with their patients was the most marked change noted. Given the pattern of interviews and investigation, at six months, for many of the couples, comparatively little progress towards a firm diagnosis and treatment had been made. The first six months were often the time when little more than initial tests would have been completed, and many couples felt that disappointingly little had happened, let alone been achieved. The emotional costs of failing to explain why this initial period was so protracted were noticeably high.

Waiting lists for the operative procedures, notably laparoscopy, meant that many of the women who needed this would have to wait at least 18 months from the time of the first appointment before it would happen. There are arguments for not doing such expensive and potentially risky procedures more quickly: some will conceive spontaneously or just with the help of general advice; others will be found to have a severe problem with the male partner. There was little evidence that trouble was taken to explain this sort of thinking to the patients, with the consequent numbers of those feeling confused and uncertain.

Some did feel clear in their understanding.

> Could not fault anyone; staff were right [= *very*] good, specially that doctor who answered all our questions, felt fairly at ease with him.
>
> (Mrs Newsome)

> I'm grateful for them explaining and not leaving us out in the cold.
>
> (Mrs Flower)

Even those who felt things had been explained in a way they could understand sometimes felt that they had to take some of the initiative in obtaining the answers they wanted.

> Very open; occasionally talked in medical terms and you had to ask what they meant – understand why it happens, but you had to ask. But they did explain. (Mr Ivy)

> No whispering behind your back. It's important your partner is there to pick up the points made; so much told to you. (Mrs Ivy)

This comment brings out the point that doctors, as much as any profession perhaps, very easily underestimate the wish for knowledge of their patients, and the need to explain technical terms or jargon. At the same time they might be forgetting the degree to which anxiety reduces the patient's ability to receive complicated messages about his or her position. As will be seen, they have a fine line to tread between talking down to their patients and assuming they can absorb or understand more than is reasonable in the circumstances. This will be highly individual.

> If you are under stress the little things matter; they could help you more if they thought a bit. Total lack of communication.   (Mr Carver)

In this context, and others quoted, comparisons can in fact be advantageous. Mrs Quick, who had a child without active treatment, noted:

> They have time to sit and listen and explain things – unlike the ante-natal clinic!

At the first follow-up interview the weight of comment was firmly against the adequacy of explanation, although, at the last, opinion seemed to be fairly evenly split. Again, they did not divide along lines of parent and childless.

> You need a chance to talk to someone who knows; you don't have the opportunity to ask anyone.   (Mr Crow)

> If someone would just take ten minutes with every patient, to explain what will happen and why; to include both husband and wife.
>
> (Mrs Crow)

A couple who had already achieved pregnancy without treatment by the time of the first follow-up complained:

> We were dissatisfied with the way the doctor treated us . . . Got the impression that the results weren't our business. 'You're just XX1234.' Didn't seem to recognise the importance of time to the couple concerned. No explanation of the time taken for the results to come through.   (Mr Coleman)

More bluntly, Mrs Green said:

> They don't explain: think we're thick.

A major factor in reducing the level of discontent seemed to be the final interview for those who were not going to be successfully treated by the Clinic. In these cases the Clinic practice was for the consultant to see the couple if possible and explain their medical status in detail. Several couples drew a clear distinction between this interview and the ones that preceded it. The couple saw an expert doctor, having a sympathetic manner, who gave them time and space fully to discuss their position.

As was noted in introducing the issues of patient satisfaction, the amount and quality of communication between patient and doctor are among the most important factors determining the feelings left behind. It is one of the most problematic to control, given that good communication requires adequate time. Fifteen-minute appointments do not facilitate this. However, it is clearly not simply a matter of time.

Waiting time

The time patients have to wait in hospital clinics is a perennial source of complaint (cf. NAHA 1987). This was certainly the case in the Infertility Clinic. The problems of staffing were clearly a significant factor, but not the only one. None of the patients reported that appointments were kept promptly. Personal observation was that attending the Clinic involved a great deal of waiting, not all unavoidable.

The practice at the time of the study is described in Chapter 5. Even when the Clinic started promptly, patients not seen first were likely to wait a considerable time beyond the appointed hour. The practice of block appointments is common, and is designed to maintain a constant 'supply' of patients for the staff. Whilst this practice does, perhaps, save valuable staff time, this study demonstrated the cost, in terms of personal anxiety and goodwill.

> Feel as if you are on a conveyor belt. They could deal with you in an appropriate manner . . . The appointments system is ridiculous; they know a lot have appointments for the same time. Doctors are cloistered from the fact that it's not always easy to get time off work. They're removed from the sharp end. Why don't they stagger them? . . . It's all bad manners. [Consultant] is treated like God. I expect appointments to be kept.
> (Mr Crow)

> It's the same as every hospital, there's another 30 have an appointment for the same time as you. Once we waited for 3½ hours and saw the doctor for 5 minutes!
> (Mr Neal)

> I didn't like the long waits in the cubicle; you get undressed and sit and sit and sit.
> (Mrs Ivy)

For some couples frustration about waiting was exacerbated by the failure of Clinic staff to keep the patients informed of delays. On several observed occasions it was known that one of the doctors would be very late, but this was not disclosed to the patients. There were also a number of occasions when the consultant was known to be absent, yet some patients who expected to see him personally were not told. Indeed, on no occasion, during the year I attended the Clinic, did a member of staff address the whole of the waiting room with information about delays, absences or any other matter, except once, to announce that the tea bar was open. One couple registered their annoyance thus:

> We just stopped going. The last appointment [with the Consultant] just never happened. Had all those appointments with different guys and had to explain it all each time . . . after three hours' wait we saw another young man . . . Could have been more honest than they were. Last visit I almost stormed out, saying 'bugger them'; we waited until 5, very nervous and very annoyed; but if he couldn't come, surely they could have told us all at 2 that he wasn't there.   (Mr Truswell)

As has been explained already, the funding situation was probably a factor, in that the ante-natal clinic and staff being used at the time were apparently not committed to the special needs of this group of patients. The move to another clinic was appreciated by those who had known both.

Problems of waiting for appointments were exacerbated for some by the lack of any camaraderie. Staff attitudes were probably a factor in this, as was the isolation and concern for confidentiality felt by many couples.

> Everyone was very quiet and separate, ill at ease. Even when we were there until 7 at night no banter started.   (Mr Truswell)

It must be a matter of concern that excessive waiting times lead to increased anxiety for the patients and to increased hostility towards the Clinic.

> At least they could tell you what is happening; you just sit and wait and see what happens. Not knowing what to expect is the worry. You can't prepare questions on the spur of the moment sometimes.
>
> (Mr Mitchell)

> Their time's valuable – what about ours? Specially when you end up with 5 minutes. It's not realistic; so much time wasting and delay.
>
> (Mr Keith)

Duration of process

The other matter of time to concern respondents was, overall, the time that investigations and any required treatment took to complete. This concern showed no sign of diminishing over the study period.

As has been discussed in some detail, there are arguments for not hurrying the process: the incidence of 'spontaneous' pregnancy; the need for several menstrual cycles to be monitored via the BBT; the time taken for hormonal treatment to affect ovulation or sperm production; the natural cycle of several weeks taken for sperm production. The problem of inadequate resources showed particularly in the 9 or 12 months' waiting lists for laparoscopy and 12 to 18 months for microsurgery obtaining at this time.

Several people did comment favourably on the pace at which the Clinic proceeded. However, two couples were comparing it favourably with a district general hospital and the third expressed a wish not to be hurried into treatment, being undecided about how far they were prepared to go.

One consequence of the failure to explain thoroughly the reasons for not increasing the pace of investigations, as well as for those factors which are simply related to inadequate resources (numbers of patients and staff, laboratory facilities), is increased frustration with what appears to be an unnecessarily protracted process.

> It seems endless; we're eager to get on with it, don't like all this waiting around. (Mr Coleman)

> Amount of time it all takes is unsettling; it would be easier if it could all be condensed in time. (Mr Truswell)

The older women were made especially anxious by the delay between appointments, being, in most cases, acutely aware of the decline of fertility with age and the rules of adoption agencies.

> I didn't think they'd let things drag on so long, for my age.
> (Mrs Grindrod)

Along with a desire to be treated by the same doctor consistently, the Crows gave the wish to speed up the whole process as the main reason for deciding to go for private care (the only couple in the study to do this).

The time taken seemed to be an abiding memory for some of the couples.

> Length of time it all takes sticks in my mind. You went one day and got an appointment for 6 weeks. You'd have taken your temperature and then you'd have to wait 6 months for the results. (Mrs Truswell)

> I'd have liked to go more often. When they said 'see you in 3 months', I thought 'that's a long time, oh no, 3 months is too long!'.
> (Mrs Mitchell)

> I always want to get on with things; the old '3 or 4 months and see how it goes' is hard. (Mr Mitchell)

The length of time that couples are in infertility treatment can be extremely long, cf. Figure 4.1. Some other patients, who did not form part of the study group, had been investigated at this and other clinics for ten years and more. The increasing sophistication of available treatments is likely, if anything, to lengthen significantly the time which couples spend under investigation.

Professor Cooke argues the value of setting finite limits to treatment wherever possible, to avoid the spectre faced by some couples of inordinately long periods of investigation with decreasing chances of success. Several couples who remained childless mentioned valuing this setting of realistic limits as helping them to come to terms with their situation. Some will, however, want to continue until every last possibility has been exhausted. From the reactions of these couples, most wanted the period of investigation to be kept as short as possible, and could see no benefits for them in the delays.

Difficult investigation

By the physical and emotional nature of the condition it is to be expected that the investigations will prove to be difficult and unpleasant, at least to some of these patients. Larger numbers might have been expected than those recorded in Table 7.2.

> He hurt me so much [internal physical examination] it put me off; put a fear of going again. But I've had them since and it's been alright.
>
> (Mrs Grindrod)

> The internals didn't allow for how tense I was, and how difficult it was to relax.   (Mrs Coleman)

In the case of Mrs Grindrod, the doctor was unable to perform the internal examination at the first appointment because she was unable to relax her muscles sufficiently. Many women would have welcomed being prepared for the internal examination. Many had not previously had to submit to this highly intrusive, and for some, embarrassing procedure. Not all, by any means, had expected it to be performed at the first appointment.

Another procedure that came in for criticism from two women was the HSG. It was described in the Clinic as a 'special' X-ray, leading them to expect it to be entirely painless, as ordinary X-rays. The introduction and passage of the radio-opaque dye can cause severe cramp.

> The HSG was very bad, terrible pain after; had to have the emergency doctor. The only warning there was was in the appointment letter.
>
> (Mrs Trafford)

One woman did, however, mention the HSG as one of the good things about her treatment, having enjoyed watching the passage of the dye through the uterus and fallopian tubes on the monitor screen.

The only investigation, other than semen analysis, performed on most of the men was the testicular biopsy. One man complained:

> The biopsy hurt. If a vasectomy is as bad, I'm having no vasectomy!
>
> (Mr Trevor)

On a more positive note, when Mr Truswell's biopsy stitching went wrong causing substantial pain, he and his wife were very pleased at the way the hospital doctor immediately travelled the 20 miles on public transport in order to rectify the problem.

A substantial level of embarrassment was admitted by these couples. Nine (30 per cent) of the men and ten (33 per cent) of the women found some aspect of the process embarrassing. The men mentioned: having female nurses in the room when being examined; the process of producing the semen sample; the Clinic being part of a women's hospital. For the women the embarrassments recalled were: the physical examination; not washing after intercourse when going for the PCT; the HSG. One woman was particularly annoyed by the indignity of the HSG: Mrs Butler described graphically how she felt, fixed in the undignified position necessary for the test, feet raised in stirrups and legs spread. She had to remain in this position for some 20 minutes, during which time the radiologist and radiographer were talking gaily about the party they had attended together.

Difficulty with the actual investigations was recalled as a problem by only a few of the couples interviewed. Since I had no reason to believe that this lack of criticism was due to reticence, this might be regarded as an achievement by the Clinic staff.

Changing doctors

This is not an uncommon complaint in the National Health Service, so the adverse reactions of these couples might be expected. Books advocating a sensitive approach to the treatment of the subfertile include this as an important matter to be avoided if possible (e.g. Winston 1986, Philipp and Carruthers 1981, Stanway 1984). The NHS traditionally appoints junior doctors on fixed length, short-term contracts. Much of the work in all specialties is undertaken by junior doctors in training, who spend only 6 months with one consultant before being moved to another post. As indicated in the description of the Clinic pattern (Chapter 5), during the period of the study the first examination, as well as much of the initial work in the Clinic, was performed by the SHO in pathology. Having an interest in infertility would be a fortunate coincidence rather than a planned factor. After seeing this doctor on the first occasion, 'return' patients would be seen either by the same doctor again, if there were not too many new patients, or one of the research workers, of whom there were several, or occasionally the senior registrar or the consultant. Remembering the 6-monthly cycle of junior registrars and the less predictable turnover of research staff, and recalling also that appointments would be spaced out with up to 3 months between, it was quite possible that a couple would never see the same doctor twice.

[There was] no continuity, we had different doctors not familiar with our case.   (Mr Dorairaj)

You should see one or two doctors maximum. Now we've seen four, and they all say something slightly different. You get confused . . . would rather cut out the middle man.   (Mr Green)

It was not simply that couples objected to a change of doctors, nor that a relationship with a particular doctor was broken, but that one never got started. It left these couples with the conviction that they did not experience a co-ordinated process as much as a series of encounters which did not successfully gel, or give them confidence that their investigation was orderly.

It's all so fast, you're never given enough time to put your view across, or talk to someone. I saw someone different each time the first three times. They don't read their own notes or believe them. On the fifth visit went back to square one with a new doctor.   (Mrs Crow)

You see a different doctor each time, he reads the notes while you are there. Not one's said the same thing! We were particularly annoyed to come back after three months and still records aren't complete and results in. If they took the trouble to read the notes before we went in, we wouldn't have felt so upset.   (Mr Keith)

Communication is only likely to improve substantially if it is possible for couples to have one or two doctors follow them right through the investigation; or if relationships with other Clinic staff can be strengthened, thus reducing the importance of continuity of the doctor.

Clinic administration

Various aspects of the organisation of the Clinic which gave concern have already been mentioned and need no repetition. This category, a quarter of the couples, made a general comment on the way in which the Clinic was organised or administered, which they felt was inadequate. None of these respondents found anything to commend in this area.

Rather annoyed by the hospital process; drawn out, too slow and casual. You get messed about.   (Mr Keith)

The main issue of organisation was the waiting and delays already discussed.

If we [his firm] provided the standard of service they do at the hospital, we'd go bankrupt in a week. But it's the only place; there's no alternative, if you blast them you get nowhere.   (Mr Crow)

If it's going to carry on they need to get their act together. The admin.
system needs sorting out. We got the impression from the nurses it was
just expected.   (Mrs Truswell)

The restricted resources available to the Clinic clearly explain some of
these shortcomings. It remains the case that the organisation of the Clinic
appeared not to give confidence to, at least, a quarter of the couples and to
create a climate of antagonism for a significant number that must undermine the work of the Clinic.

Husband left out

One aspect of the procedure of the Clinic that caused concern to several
couples, and seemed not to have been properly explained, was the reason
for continuing to investigate the woman, even to the point of laparoscopy,
where the only deficit identified was in the man. It is argued in the
textbooks (e.g. Philipp and Carruthers 1981) that it would be unwise to put
couples through the difficult experience of DI or IVF unless you could be
fairly sure that the woman was fertile enough to stand a good chance of
success. The couples in this study felt they had been left to draw this
conclusion for themselves.

It's not fair going through that laparoscopy when they know what the
problem is.   (Mrs Turner)

Although there are good scientific reasons for the more extensive investigation of the female to achieve a baseline assessment, it can reinforce an
impression that the Clinic is simply content, for sexist reasons, to expect
more investment by the woman regardless of the nature of the problems.

As with so many infertility services, the one studied here could not rely
on the active and enthusiastic co-operation of a urology service where male
problems were encountered: varicocele ligation involved a waiting list of
two years. Only two infertility services were run at this time in the whole of
Great Britain by urologists. One of the most recent medical texts on male
infertility is written by a gynaecologist (Jequier 1986). One might infer an
unconscious historical sexism amongst clinicians, researchers, and patients,
in the slow advance of knowledge about male fertility and its deficits,
which leads to this apparent differential attention.

Some men did say that they wanted to play a fuller part than they felt
allowed to do, although it was interesting to note that none still articulated
this view at the final interview. This might be another facet of that tendency
amongst the men, already noted, to put the experience firmly to one side
when no longer attending the Clinic.

I felt excluded; I only got to talk to the tea lady! . . . I resent being ignored totally. I was only asked to give a sample by the wife being given a bottle. I would have expected to have been included in the interviews. I've never even seen the doctor, let alone been interviewed.

(Mr Crow)

In a social climate which still more readily focuses on the woman when a partnership is infertile, an infertility clinic will need to make a conscious effort to engage the men fully in the investigation. This Clinic began to make changes, partly as a result of this study bringing certain issues to light, e.g. the wording of the appointment letter. The change of clinic location made an impact. More needed to be done, however, to reduce those obstacles within the control of the hospital to men's fuller participation.

Consultant not seen

As in any specialist medical referral it is to be expected that, when referred to a consultant, the patient is likely to set store on seeing him or her and feel somewhat let down if always seen by a junior doctor. An undercurrent of such concern was found amongst these couples, who had either not seen the consultant at all or only on one occasion. This experience is, of course, common in the NHS, given patterns of consultant referral and appointment. The pattern in the Clinic was for junior doctors to undertake the 'work-up' and initial investigations and only at a later stage, for more complex problems or for a 'turning point' interview, would the consultant see the patients. By 'turning point' I mean the appointment at which couples, for whom the standard treatments had produced no result, faced important choices. These might include DI, or complex, relatively unsuccessful, time- and emotion-demanding treatments like IVF and tubal microsurgery which could also involve a long wait. The consultant felt that it was fairer to such couples to present them with an assessment of their realistic chances of success as well as the demands that going further would place upon them. He or she felt, humanely, that infertile couples were sometimes encouraged by the enthusiasm of doctors to become obsessed with more and more treatment in the face of ever-diminishing chances of a pregnancy. For a large number of the couples, whether or not they had decided to continue, this interview was remembered as being very helpful. The Crows, who were otherwise so critical, regarded this discussion as the only good thing about their attendance at the Clinic.

If you saw the top man more often you wouldn't mind so much.

(Mrs Mitchell)

Abortions

People with a fertility problem might be expected to find abortion upsetting. Unfortunately for these patients, and probably for most infertility
patients at any hospital, part of the overall task of an obstetrics and gynaecology service is the termination of unwanted pregnancies. Several couples
recounted the distress they suffered on this account.

The problem arose here with in-patient treatment, usually the laparoscopy which required a stay of several days, being conducted under general
anaesthetic. Whilst the consultant told me that it was policy to segregate the
two groups of women wherever possible, it was either not always possible
or sometimes forgotten.

> Having two girls in for abortion at the same time made it very
> distressing.   (Mrs Flower)

> At the time of the first operation, a girl in the next room was in for an
> abortion. I found that very hard. They should put them in a different
> ward. It's a horrible feeling, knowing what they're in for, and what
> you're in for. Another time I was put near to the pregnant women and
> you could hear the babies crying at night. They should try to separate
> you.   (Mrs Holt)

In a situation of limited resources and pressures on hospital beds and
operating facilities, it might be very difficult to avoid such conflicts.
However, it is clearly essential that staff should be sensitive to the feelings
of both infertile and aborting women.

Two instances of appalling insensitivity were recounted in the course of
these interviews; the first by one of the women interviewed in preparation
for the main study. An aborting woman was 4 months pregnant when
talking to my respondent who was waiting to go for a laparoscopy. Pointing
to her stomach and making a throat-cutting gesture, the woman was
reported to have said:

> Let this little parasite wait – I'm getting rid of him tomorrow!

A less excusable experience was that of the Newsomes, who had a child by
the time of this comment:

> One thing I found terrible was having women on the same landing
> having abortions. I don't think they should put infertile women and those
> having abortions together, that's cruel. I begged to go early because of
> that. I was waiting for my husband to come, and the person who was
> taking my bed was in for an abortion. I'm not anti-abortion, but that's
> awful. It shouldn't be like that; it hurts even now. I actually saw a fetus

in a jar in Sister's office! I asked her if it was from an abortion; 'yes', she
says.   (Mrs Newsome)

There was one on the game [i.e. a prostitute] having an abortion, who
was going back on the game that night.   (Mr Newsome)

These poignant recollections point to a source of distress which could to a
large extent be avoided, given the sensitivity of all staff to the situation,
even if only by warning the childless patients.

Privacy

An aspect of the stigma felt by so many couples was the desire to preserve
their privacy.

Several people mentioned their dislike of having results conveyed to
them with groups of students present. This was particularly likely to happen
during in-patient investigations.

Those who underwent DI were naturally concerned to preserve the
confidentiality of their treatment, as none intended broadcasting the fact, or
registering the birth in the then legally prescribed way, as 'father unknown'.

It could do with being a bit more secretive. When you go in you sit
waiting and someone you know could see you. If people see you going
to a DI clinic they start putting two and two together.   (Mr Trevor)

When he told him [of his azoospermia] all the nurses and students were
in; it wasn't private enough . . . Thought it would be a bit more private;
it's a bit casual.   (Mrs Trevor)

When we were told my results . . . well I can take bad news. My wife
started crying; we objected to having two student doctors sitting there
when we were given the news. They'd no right to be there then. It's not
nice for others to know.   (Mr Carver)

This is a dilemma, not confined to infertility, which faces all teaching
hospitals. Students need to learn; and, arguably, medical education is still
poor at teaching students the human side of medicine and how to handle
emotionally difficult situations. However, these objectives have to be
reconciled by the careful seeking of consent from patients who might feel
they are being asked to expose very private parts of their lives to public
view. Some of these patients did not feel their consent was sought.

IMPROVING THE SERVICE

Attention to the problems outlined in detail above would contribute substantially to an overall improvement in the emotional quality and impact of the infertility service. Respondents made a number of suggestions of specific changes that they would like to see implemented.

Some involved the location and facilities of the hospital. Parking on an inner city site was difficult. Until the latter part of the study period there were no refreshment facilities. The Clinic itself was not comfortably furnished, and the cubicles in which women had to wait after changing to see the doctor were isolated and bare. The frustration with waiting had therefore been fuelled by sitting for long periods in a fairly uncongenial situation. The frustration with changing doctors, and the length of time waiting, indicated the need for better staffing.

Two issues were raised of particular interest to this study. Firstly, in different ways, nine couples (32 per cent) identified the need for counselling, better information or self-help groups. Secondly, more consideration of the husband in the process was felt important by eight couples (29 per cent).

Personal support

As has been noted, there was considerable concern at the limited opportunities to talk through the nature of the fertility problems they faced, their feelings and the solutions which were proposed. The lack of adequate information and explanation headed the list of concerns. Apart from consultation with the doctor, no opportunities of this sort were available in the Clinic at this time.

The nursing staff saw their role as ensuring the availability of patients, with their notes, for the doctor, testing urine samples, measuring height and weight, chaperoning during physical examinations of female patients by male doctors, and instruction in BBT charts. They rarely appeared to get involved in talking to the patients in more general terms, unless a patient approached them with a query. (It should be remembered that this changed with the move to the gynaecology out-patients clinic.) There was certainly no attempt to talk to patients about what they might be feeling, or to help them understand the procedures of the Clinic or what the doctor might do or say. None of these patients had any positive comments to make about the nursing service in the Clinic itself, although several subsequently commended the attention given by the nurses in the new clinic and during hospital in-patient stays.

Social work support to the Infertility Clinic was discussed with the two social workers successively responsible for this service during the course of the study. In common with much medical social work (Butrym and Horder 1983, Davidson and Clarke 1989) this service was primarily reactive to the needs identified by the referring medical staff. In the case of the Infertility Clinic, this was perceived as a setting in which there were substantial problems of the sort social workers are most sensitive to, and skilled in helping. However, very few referrals were received, and those which were did not always seem appropriate to the social worker.

The social workers perceived the patients as having a significant need for counselling and supportive casework, but as commanding a lesser priority than other demands by other doctors. In discussion, the general level of pain and anxiety amongst these patients was noted, as well as the aspects of the hospital service, not specific to the Infertility Clinic, which exacerbated their distress.

The patients who were referred fell, mainly, into three categories;

1. Patients for whom no more can be done, who have been advised to discuss adoption.
2. DI applicants about whom medical staff have substantial reservations.
3. Patients for whom no more can be done, who, in the doctor's opinion, appear to have difficulty in accepting this.

The social workers had some concern that doctors might on occasion, with the more distressed patients, be tempted to ask the social worker to 'break the bad news' of there being little that could be offered in the way of treatment, and little hope of their conceiving.

Although exact figures were not available, it was estimated that the demand for service from the Infertility Clinic was only some three patients a year. Several hundred referrals were received from other sources in a year, many of these from the multi-disciplinary in-patient ward rounds. The infertility service being primarily focused on out-patients, plus short-stay investigative admissions, was a structural reason for the infertility service having a lower demand profile than other services for which the social workers were responsible. The social workers, therefore, felt unable to 'go looking' for work in this area.

None of the couples in this study had been referred to a hospital social worker. Those who applied to adopt, which is considered in the next chapter, were seen by social workers from an adoption agency; in every case, their local social services department. Those who went forward for DI were counselled prior to acceptance.

For some couples, the view that infertility has a major psychological component was firmly in mind. It should be said that the Clinic did nothing overtly to support this belief. The view of the consultant matched that developed in the review of the literature in Chapter 2. Whilst there are important emotional consequences of infertility, there is little evidence that a significant proportion of infertility is primarily psychological in origin. Several couples contrasted their understanding that psychological causes could be important with the apparent lack of interest in such matters at the Clinic.

> It's all so impersonal; but it's an emotional problem. Absolutely no consideration is given to the emotional side of it. Feel as if you're on a conveyor belt . . . I feel infertility is 90 per cent psychological; from documentary programmes, magazine articles that impression is put across strongly; therefore it's insensitive, building another barrier.
>
> (Mr Crow)

> They don't seem to investigate the psychological aspects at all; but I think it affects infertility. Some people could be very tense and they don't seem to consider this. Don't most doctors have some training in the emotional side of infertility? They just looked at the physical side. Someone trained in that side would help someone suffering from depression, for instance.
>
> (Mr Dorairaj)

Just as there were differing views of the helpfulness of talking about problems as a means of coping with them (see Chapter 5) so the suggestion that counselling should be available was not a general view. The idea of compulsory counselling is to some extent a contradiction in terms. However, it did emerge that it should be readily available in such a clinic, both as a direct service and for the indirect contribution it could make to general practice.

There are, of course, gender issues in this context. Studies for the National Marriage Guidance Council (see, e.g., Hunt 1985) and Brannen and Collard (1982) agree that in marital counselling men are less likely to make the first contact, seek help alone or continue with counselling. O'Brien sums up the general concern that men are often peripheral in counselling.

Reference to the value that couples saw in talking to me about their experiences was the most frequent way in which counselling was raised.

> I like talking to someone about all this; there's only my daughter and Hannah (you know her too don't you?*) and you that I've talked to, and it does help to talk things over.
>
> (Mrs Holt)

---

* Mrs Holt and Mrs Flower independently discovered they had each been interviewed for this study; this was the only instance I came across of a friendship developing between patients.

There was no opportunity to talk to anyone, discuss the problem properly, as we are talking to you now.   (Mr Young)

We've not talked to anyone together at any stage, only you. It would help to have someone like you at the hospital. We'd have liked an initial explanation and if they'd got to know us a bit better. Someone's needed to explain everything.   (Mrs Lamb)

As my role in the interviews was entirely one of encouraging them to discuss their views and listening carefully, this presumably was the contribution they valued. Evidence of the importance many of these couples attached to the opportunity that my interview had given them to discuss the whole process came in some surprising ways. At the final interview, some three years later, there was an extraordinarily clear recollection of the earlier interviews I had conducted. In two cases the unremarkable way I take coffee was remembered; in a third it was recalled that I did not smoke, although neither issue had assumed any apparent importance at the earlier interviews.

The value of a self-help group was less often articulated. Only six couples had even vaguely heard of one of the voluntary associations concerned with the welfare of childless people: the 'National Association for the Childless' and 'Child'. In two cases only the wife had heard of one. In no case could they name an organisation. The Infertility Clinic seemed to be uncertain of the value of such a group at the time. Although the consultant was sympathetic, literature supplied did not seem to appear in the Clinic. Nursing staff showed no interest in the idea. One couple reported asking the nursing staff if there was anything, and was told there was no such organisation. Only two couples directly rejected the idea.

Not considered it; it's only for people it affects very strongly.

(Mr David)

Can't see the point; it won't get you a baby!   (Mrs David)

We don't consider ourselves childless.   (Mr Turner)

The case for such organisations was put by Mr Carver:

Who can you talk to about this? We elected not to talk to our friends. If there was an organisation for infertile people like AA, it would help. Every couple who go should be told there are organisations like that. It wouldn't do any harm to talk to strangers. Sure, most people want the secret side, but wouldn't spoil it to have somebody to talk to.

(Mr Carver)

It is interesting to note the emphasis on secrecy here; the common perception that being infertile was a discreditable feature akin to alcoholism. Mrs Newsome echoed these feelings:

> I think there should be somewhere you can go to talk to someone about it, who's been through it. An association for it. It's not something you talk to everyone about. It's not a nice thing to admit . . . it would be nice to talk to others in the same boat and compare feelings. You don't know how others feel. (Mrs Newsome)

There was one instance in which a belief in emotional causes of infertility might have been seriously misleading treatment by discouraging the necessary rigour in identifying contributory factors.

> Sure we were right to go; we did get some results showing no problems which must have helped the psychology anyway. Our own doctor mentioned the probability of it being psychological before referring us. Can't remember if the hospital used the expression. I think it was perhaps more me. I get tense very easily. The blood pressure only got down to normal levels recently. (Mr Monk)

Mr Monk was being treated for depression and hypertension, and the medication for both conditions can depress sperm quality. It was suspected that Mrs Monk had an ovulatory problem which was treated empirically. When he was no longer being treated, they conceived.

The availability of a service in the Clinic which could provide counselling, facilitate self-help in groups and ensure that the emotional needs of the patients were fully acknowledged would strengthen this infertility service considerably. The Human Fertilisation and Embryology Act 1990 has since required that all infertility clinics provide counselling services.

Involvement of the men

In the discussion of complaints about the service were noted those husbands who felt that they had not been fully included in the process. There were others who had been little involved and who did not see this as a difficulty. In contrast to the advice in the literature and the stated philosophy of the Clinic, there was little evidence of a conscious effort to include and involve the husbands. The evidence discussed above suggests that ensuring men's full involvement is likely to require specific measures.

From the start, the orientation of the Clinic appeared to be towards the woman. The appointment card was addressed to her, offering a gynaecological appointment at a women's hospital which made no mention of the man. One aspect of this orientation was the siting of the Infertility Clinic in the ante-natal clinic of a women's hospital (a financial expedient, it should be noted). Four couples particularly complained about this perceived insensitivity.

> The worst part was, you're extremely psychologically disturbed by the infertility, yet it's set in a clinic full of pregnant women. [*Parentcraft class at same time*.] That's extremely insensitive, since you're wanting children, you're conscious of seeing so many children – doesn't help at all.
> (Mr Crow)

> I remember the ante-natal (or was it the post-natal?) clinic was the same place. That would really affect you, and all those posters on the walls; it was a bit heartless.
> (Mrs Truswell)

When the Clinic moved to the gynaecology out-patients some time after the recruitment of this sample was completed, several couples mentioned that it felt much more congenial.

Junior medical staff seemed to pursue their own inclinations concerning the involvement of patients' partners; the consultant's policy was that the woman should be asked if her partner was present. If he was he should be examined and asked to provide a semen sample; if he was not, his wife would be asked to transmit the request for a sample and ask him to attend on the next occasion. In practice, even if he was there, the partner was often ignored. If he was not present, provided there was no deficit in his semen analysis, he was not always invited to attend. Some husbands managed never to attend the Clinic, without this apparently affecting the course of treatment.

This approach was implicitly welcomed by some of the men.

> It never occurred to me to go. I've had no direct communication; they gave Myra the results. I've never discussed sperm production with any of the doctors. I wasn't surprised at not being involved; I've not felt excluded. I would have gone if they'd asked me to, or if Myra had wanted. You're never sure who will be seen anyway, so it could be a waste of time.
> (Mr Butler)

> I didn't know much about it. Never actually went with her or took her for any of the tests . . . It never occurred to me that I could or should have been more involved.
> (Mr Carter)

However, there were others who were unhappy at being given the impression that they were peripheral to the whole exercise.

> My only contact was when I took my sample – it was taken off me by the

porter! and no feedback, not a postcard with the result, not even a
receipt! (Mr Keith)

I just don't feel involved. I'm kept in the dark; just get to hear about
things second hand. (Mr Lamb)

I feel totally excluded; always left in the waiting room. No-one else said a
word to you. I resented their apparent lack of interest in me. (Mr Crow)

It is worth noting that Mr Lamb had a normal sperm count. The sense of being
ignored had nothing to do with whether or not there was a male problem. The
Clinic, therefore, reinforced the tendency noted elsewhere that even where the
fertility deficit was on the man's part the women seemed to carry a disproportionate amount of the emotional burden this imposed.

The burden of carrying the communication with the Clinic was also
noted as a reason for involving the men more.

I just took the sample in; not involved. It could have helped if I'd been
there too; if one misunderstands, the other could help. I thought they
were only bothered to see the one they were concerned with; the one that
needed treatment . . . Can't see why both couldn't go in at the same time.
Can't say I tried to get in; there's an air of 'it's our responsibility, we'll
do what's needed'. There's got to be that, but can't there be an attitude
of let's talk to both of them and see them? (Mr Flower)

More evidence was noted in this connection of the extent to which women
seemed prepared to protect their husbands, and take on the responsibility.

It was her appointment, but I wouldn't have gone anyway. Nothing to do
with me, it wasn't even mentioned. (Mr Keith)

It was then revealed by Mrs Keith that the doctor had asked her to bring him in
with her; she had not passed on the message. Mr Keith seemed surprised at this.

I didn't realise I would be wanted; could have gone, but the wife said
'don't bother'. (Mr Mitchell)

He wasn't at all keen on giving a sample. I took it in. He was em-
barrassed about it. (Mrs Menzies)

The case of the Mitchells has been mentioned in this context before, as the
clearest example of a man denying totally his involvement, with which his
wife colluded. One exchange illustrated this:

I can't take him showing his disappointment. I can manage my own. I
felt more of a failure with him getting too involved with it. I don't know
what's next . . . (Mrs Mitchell)

. . . the patter of tiny feet I expect!   (Mr Mitchell)

I don't know why he's so optimistic.   (Mrs Mitchell)

I've not felt the involved party. I'm normal at least.   (Mr Mitchell)

Mrs Mitchell did have several problems, but Mr Mitchell was severely oligospermic, which did not prevent Mrs Mitchell saying, 'He's not really the problem.' They subsequently had a child by DI which they insisted to me was naturally conceived.

It would be wrong to give the impression that all of the husbands readily left the responsibility entirely with their wives. However, the contrary examples were in a clear minority.

I was keen to come every time.   (Mr Ivy)

I always went with her; it was a joint thing. It was our problem and we went through it together.   (Mr Neal)

These couples made it plain that the social attitudes which place the weight of expectation on women to bear children for their husbands are still very real. Neither the Infertility Clinic nor the wives, whatever the intention expressed, appeared able to put the same expectations of involvement on the men. If men did get involved wholeheartedly, this was a matter for note and gratitude from their wives. Even when so many men stated that their wives were more upset by the childlessness, this did not encourage them to offer more support than they themselves wished with the Clinic appointments. The clear impression was that the Clinic had low expectations of the men's involvement, and these are largely shared by their wives.

ROLE OF THE GP

The importance of the GP's role in relation to people getting into the infertility system in the first place has been discussed in Chapter 5. For most people, it seems that the decision to consult the GP about failure to conceive is an important step, which is not taken lightly. Many seem to delay substantially before this move. As appeared in the GPS, a not insignificant proportion may never take that step, choosing instead to accept their situation without challenge.

It is now important to consider the continuing role the GP played during the course of investigation, as well as the views on this matter of the GPs responding to the Family Practitioner Study.

A consistently positive view was recorded by the study group. At both initial and final interviews almost half of the men and two-thirds of the women replied that their GP had been 'quite/very sympathetic' in his or her attitude to their difficulties. Only at the first completion were answers 'quite/very unsympathetic' given – by two men and two women (7 per cent). (The difference between the proportions of men and women is explained by their being more than a quarter of the men who had not consulted their own doctors about the infertility.) The GPs questioned saw an important role for themselves in supporting their patients and the activities of the hospital.

Although there was a very small number of those who appeared to see no role for themselves once the referral for specialist investigation had been made, it is interesting to note that single-handed doctors and those aged over 40 were twice as likely to give this answer as those who were in partnership, or were younger. The younger GPs favoured counselling and support, and the older ones advice and explanation. This probably reflects changing attitudes to the relationship between doctor and patient, but may also reflect a simple change of semantics, whereby 'counselling' could mean the same as 'advice'. If these two categories are considered together, then 71.2 per cent of all GPs would see themselves as offering one of these forms of help.

One doctor emphasised the importance of explanations:

Hospital tends to blind patients with science. (#42)

The essence of counselling and support was expressed by another as:

Interpreter and friend. (#25)

The sense of caring for the interests of the 'whole' patient gave the idea of liaison more than a passive connotation for one doctor.

Prevent over-enthusiastic treatment with poor success rates; generally monitor the situation. (#124)

Table 7.3 GP's role during investigation (FPS)

	No. [1]	%
Counselling/support	82	61.7
Advice/explanation	57	42.9
Medical assistance/supervision	20	15.0
Liaison	7	5.3
Nil	15	11.3

1. N=133; multiple replies gives totals in excess of 100 per cent.

When Clinic patients were asked their views of the part in their investigation played by their GPs, a slightly less positive view emerged. Fourteen (50 per cent) expressed positive views, five (18 per cent) negative and nine (32 per cent) neutral, pointing out that he or she had played no significant part.

Amongst the positive views were:

> He was very supportive and helpful; took an interest, and sent us early, even though we'd only been trying six months. Glad he did; consultant said our GP was on the ball to send us so early.   (Mrs Ivy)

They were not always well placed to liaise as information could be slow reaching the GP. Showing interest was still appreciated:

> He didn't get the results for us; asked if we'd heard owt [= *anything*].
>   (Mr Young)

> He's kept asking; been concerned.   (Mrs Young)

The GPs' efforts to keep in touch with progress and help their patients understand what was going on, if necessary, was appreciated, thus filling the gap left by any failure of the Clinic in this respect.

> She allayed a lot of our fears by explaining the results, and what she should do.   (Mrs Mitchell)

> Great! 'Anytime you want to talk about anything, come and see me,' he said.   (Mr Thurston)

Those unhappy with the GP's contribution were a smaller group. One issue was the readiness with which the doctor referred on for specialist investigation. Mrs Neal, one of the otherwise satisfied patients, noted that she 'had to have a row with him to get referred'. One couple had very bad feelings towards their own GP's locum:

> This locum gave us the results of his test with the comment 'you're sterile so you can't have any children. There's nothing else that can be done for you.' Very offhand; that was thoroughly unprofessional conduct in our mind – first we knew of it!   (Mr Carver)

As emphasised in the discussion of the explanations given by the Clinic doctors, it is important to remember, in considering such comments, the feelings of the patients receiving the information. These might well lead to misunderstandings of substance and attitude. By the same token, the feelings of the doctor about having to convey such bad news might hinder him or her in giving the news in the most sensitive way possible. A locum who does not know the patient is not well placed to undertake such a task.

A similar concern was expressed in relation to a group practice, where the couple felt that the doctors knew so little about the patients that the service they gave, perhaps inevitably, felt distanced and impersonal.

In the FPS the GPs were asked what, in their view, were the specific problems presented or created by patients with a fertility deficit (Table 7.4).

Slightly over half of those doctors replying felt that such patients presented particular issues that required a thoughtful response. Half of the doctors under 40 years of age felt that these patients required support because of their anxiety, as opposed to a quarter of the older GPs. Comparing these answers by the sex of the GP, half of the women GPs gave this answer, but only one-third of the men. The five GPs who described these patients in negative terms, as demanding or difficult, were all men. This might be taken as some support for a view that younger, particularly female, doctors are especially sensitive to the emotional component of childlessness for their patients.

The most frequent reply was that they presented no particular problems.

> Generally they are good partners, caring for each other. Present no problem.   (#120)

Several doctors noted no evidence of major psychological problems:

> In my previous practice, childlessness was not associated with a higher level of depression and psychoneurotic illness.   (#27)

Of those feeling that there were problems of anxiety and the need for support from the doctor, the following are typical replies:

> They are usually upset and worried and find one or two years' delay at the Infertility Clinic very trying.   (#36)

> It is important to relieve guilt and help the couple accept infertility if the treatment does not work.   (#39)

Table 7.4 Specific problems of subfertile patients (FPS)

	No. [1]	%
Nil	44	46.3
Anxiety/require support	32	33.7
Need time	6	6.3
Demanding/difficult	5	5.3
Other/combined answer	8	8.4

1. *N*=95; missing cases=38.

Often it can need a lot of psycho-social support and counselling, which
is not easy to give or accept.   (#120)

In a context in which it appears to be accepted that short consultations are
the norm, it is not surprising that some doctors should be concerned that
these patients need more of their time than many others.

Need time as they often have inadequate knowledge of their own physi-
ology and are referred too soon or over-investigated, without adequate
explanation.   (#14)

Few of the doctors appeared to have negative images of such patients,
notwithstanding the level of criticism directed at GPs in this study. Such
negative comments as were offered by the doctors suggested that these
patients tended to have unrealistic expectations, or could not accept a
negative result, always wanting to try another doctor, or being impatient.
The overall picture was one of substantial concern for the special needs of
these people, without their being generally seen as 'neurotic' or
'demanding'.

This picture was reinforced in the responses to the question concerning
the priority such patients enjoyed; 72.9 per cent thought the priority given
was 'about right', 10.9 per cent that it was 'rather high' or 'too high', and
16.3 per cent 'rather low' or 'too low'. In a climate of ever-increasing
demands for scarce medical resources, particularly controversial at the time
of this study when it was widely believed that NHS resources were inadequate, it is a measure of the concern of these GPs that only 1 in 10 felt that
the subfertile were getting more than a fair share of resources. Again,
single-handed and male doctors were more likely to feel this than other
groups of GPs. It was interesting that one GP commented:

We seem to get a good service, but I expect, country-wide, it is not so
adequate; also expectations are low – it's all so new.   (#7)

It is not intended to imply that all those who felt that the infertile received
a higher priority than was justified were unsympathetic to their plight.
Priorities are clearly a major dilemma in relation to the allocation of scarce
resources in any area of medicine. One doctor anticipated this:

I sympathise with the individual suffering infertility causes, but I feel it
should not be a priority when considering the overall health problems of
the community.   (#12)

Another GP hinted at the dilemma in his practice, in oblique terms:

Subfertility is not a problem; hyperfertility is!   (#58)

Recent publicity about developments has focused on the dramatic, high-technology treatments; prompting one doctor to comment:

> If medical resources deteriorate further, then this ought to be an area to receive cuts before other parts of the service.   (#39)

The question of priorities did prompt a number of GPs to raise the very difficult issues of how the needs of this group can be weighed against those of, for instance, the disabled and elderly. For a number of doctors the relative claims of abortion and subfertility on the budgets of the health service came in for comment.

> They deserve any help that can be given as they have got equal rights for their needs as others who seek urgent help asking for abortions.   (#68)

The concentration on resources in these comments was on those of the hospital services rather than GPs.

> I tend to regard all but the basic management of subfertility as a specialist pastime. This view also seems to be held by the gynaecologists. I have had no personal experience of handling the psychological impact of infertility; perhaps my lot are stoical or else the clinics deal with their psyche [*sic*] problems.   (#105)

As has been discussed in relation to the Clinic couples, there could be a danger of the contribution of GPs, and indeed their nursing colleagues, becoming devalued by the glamour of modern developments.

> This problem is best dealt with in the setting of the family practice, and every support should be given for this. It should not be a separate item, cut off from other problems and the GP should be involved at all stages of specialist examination as he has the continuing care of the family.
> (#86)

There is clearly a valuable role in basic reproductive advice for those who might still need specialist help, but also for those who remain 'hidden' and unwilling to seek hospital treatment. The GP is in the best position to give this sort of advice and help, with his or her (often) longer term knowledge of the individual patient and his or her social and family context. Other studies (e.g. Cartwright and Anderson 1981) have shown the extent to which the family doctor is still seen as a valued confidant. The management of infertility is certainly one of the areas in which the GP has an essential part to play, which can facilitate the interventions of the hospital services.

SUMMARY

There were substantial areas of concern about the service provided by the Infertility Clinic, but also many positive feelings. In comparison with other general studies of patient satisfaction, it seemed that these patients were less satisfied. Both the complaints and the compliments seemed to diminish over time. Those who remained childless were no more critical than those who had children; and those who had children little more positive.

It is a matter of regret that some of the difficulties recounted by the patients seemed to cloud the whole experience and their feelings towards the staff. It was encouraging to note that some of the factors within the control of the staff were improved during the course of the study. It is very likely that many infertility services elsewhere are still unimproved in those regards.

The gender differentials in the service were noted; in part these simply reflect prevalent social mores. Whilst it is the case that the burden of infertility falls unfairly on women, an important contribution of an infertility service could be in the efforts it makes to encourage the sharing of this burden.

These couples gave strong evidence of the demand for closer attention to their needs for personal support and opportunities to share their distress. Jones (1991) and, in the context of miscarriage, Moulder (1990) both emphasise the crucial importance of hospital staff being able to acknowledge fully the emotional needs of their patients who are undergoing deeply distressing experiences for which strictly medical solutions are inadequate. Improvements in communication, at both practical and emotional levels, are urgently needed.

Family doctors played very little part in the treatment of these people. On the whole they were regarded favourably by their patients, who would prefer their GPs to take a more active role. The interest of the doctors replying to the FPS questionnaire was itself encouraging. Naturally, those who replied might be expected to include the more interested; but they were 51 per cent of the population of GPs. Although GPs would no doubt find it hard to commit more time to this particular problem, it seemed that for the health service as a whole, this might lead to a better and more efficient service for the subfertile.

8   Resolving childlessness

Patients attending an infertility clinic are naturally looking to resolve their childlessness by having a child. As has been seen, this road is not open to all; in this study 16 (53 per cent) had a child during the course of the study, three (10 per cent) as a result of DI (donor insemination). In addition, a child was placed for adoption with one of the couples and another couple fostered several children. At the final interview 13 (43 per cent) were still without children. Some of these childless couples were having to make firm deci- sions about a future without children.

The concern of this chapter is to consider the experiences of the four main avenues aside from continuing in treatment: remaining childless; children; DI; adoption.

THE ALTERNATIVES

Having no choice: this was one of the most common ways of describing the feeling of involuntary childlessness; it involved the loss of one of the most fundamental and taken-for-granted choices, the bearing of children.

Some of the couples were anxious to hold on to control of one area of choice; how far they went in treatment in the hope of a birth. The rapid development of treatments for infertility during the period of this research made available various new stratagems. Without exception, these new approaches involved the couple, particularly the woman, in giving more and more time and energy, both physical and emotional, in the pursuit of a child. The point at which to decide that the costs outweighed the likely increased chance of pregnancy became an important issue for some of those still in treatment at the final interview. As mentioned already, some couples started the process with strong feelings about not 'getting sucked in too far'.

At both interviews the couples were asked about the alternatives they would consider if they were unsuccessful in having their own children (Table 8.1). (*N.B.* This was an open question about alternatives, not a series of closed questions about the options presented here.) Three had already become pregnant at the second interview, and 16 by the last.

Not surprisingly, adoption was the single most considered possibility, notwithstanding the general appreciation of just how difficult it is to be accepted to adopt. 'You have to be spotless, perfect' as one couple put it, rather despairingly. It is also clear that DI was not initially on the agenda for many couples. Inevitably, the couples replying to this question at the final interview were in a position in which it was necessary that they had considered the alternatives to having their own children; the matter was pressed upon them by the sense of 'closing doors' and by the Clinic doctors as part of the 'counselling' process involved at the later stages.

At the final interview, six (21 per cent) were continuing in treatment or were on waiting lists for further treatment. One couple was waiting for DI; three were on the IVF waiting lists (including Mrs Holt who was removed several days later); two were being given hormone therapy. In addition, two couples were considering returning for further help having borne one child as a result of treatment and wishing to have a second child, without thus far having any success on their own.

The couples waiting for IVF were all quite sceptical of their chances of success. Each described it as the final chance, and seemed to have no illusions that, at this time particularly, this was 'the least successful of all treatments' (Winston 1986), notwithstanding sensationalist media publicity, and the enthusiasm of its pioneers, Steptoe and Edwards and subsequent promoters. The IVF programme was just starting at this hospital

Table 8.1 Alternatives couples were prepared to consider

	FU1				FU2			
	Consider [1]	%	Not [2]	%	Consider	%	Not	%
Adoption	15	60	4	13	15	75	4	20
Fostering	3	12	2	8	5	25	5	25
DI	2	8	1	4	6	30	5	25
Childfree	7	28	0	0	3	15	0	0
None	4	16	13	52	0	0	0	0
Total	N = 25				N = 20			

N.B. Totals exceed those responding due to multiple replies.
1. Would consider this option.
2. Would not consider this option.
Compare with Table 4.8: Outcomes.

at the time of the final interviews in 1984/5. It was being offered on a private, and highly selective, basis in the University Clinic at a cost subsidised by the Clinic which has charitable status (£400 per treatment). It seemed that the Clinic was giving these women a realistic picture of their chances of giving birth to a child in this way. No births had yet occurred in this programme, although they were to do so not long afterwards.

The two women receiving hormone pump therapy saw this also as the final chance.

> In our own mind we've written it off . . . Nothing's going to happen.
> (Mrs Crow)

> We're just guinea pigs . . . we'll try anything. (Mrs Lamb)

Mrs Lamb was the only one of the six still in treatment who would pursue anything that was suggested. Most were much more cautious.

> I'm 38 now – don't want to build up my hopes again. Not sure how long I'll keep going. (Mrs Holt)

At the final interview all the couples were asked if they had any regrets about embarking upon investigations of their infertility. Only two said that they did in some ways regret the step. Those who had children might not be expected to have such regrets, but even those who were not successfully treated felt that it had been the correct thing to do.

Those who did regret being referred to the Clinic (one still childless, the other with a child) replied in terms of having felt themselves lose control over the process. Stanway (1984) characterises this as like the feeling of being on a merry-go-round. The metaphor of the treadmill might be more appropriate for some of the couples interviewed in this study (Monach 1985).

> It carries you away. We went along to find out [why], not just to get pregnant. (Mrs Keith)

> You get caught up in it, and carried along. (Mr Keith)

> Yes, I do! Not long after the miscarriage, I said to me mother 'I'd never have started, if I knew what I do now'. (Mrs Holt)

It might be that an infertility clinic sometimes underestimates the primary concern of some couples simply to ensure that there is no significant pathology preventing conception. Even if no child was born, eliminating the worry of major problems was in itself valued.

> No. Apart from anything else the endometriosis has been treated which can get very serious. That's one thing to get out. (Mrs Lamb)

Some who had not had a child naturally felt the disappointment, particularly if there had not been a conclusive diagnosis of the problem.

> Bit of a waste of time; not got a conclusion. (Mr Dorairaj)

The great majority felt, however, that whatever the problems they had experienced or complaints they had, it had been worth while.

> Glad I went through it; makes me feel at least I tried. Don't regret it.
> (Mrs Trafford)

> Some good might come of it; even if it only helps someone else.
>
> (Mrs Kitchen)

> No; answered a few questions. We might have blamed each other if we didn't go. (Mr Trevor)

For all the complaints and personal distress which were registered in these interviews, the couples very largely felt that they took the correct decision in being referred to the Infertility Clinic.

More than half of both the men and women interviewed, whether childless or parent, agreed that children are important to a marriage. Similarly, amongst those who answered that children are not important to a marriage, some had children and some remained childless. Therefore, the childless did not all adopt a firm rationalisation of denial. Mrs Holt was the only childless woman to link marriage and children firmly.

> Children make a marriage really. It's alright to wait a year or two to get straight, but after that they make a marriage. Probably that's what's depressing us. I can't imagine a marriage without children. I'm not sure what he thinks, we haven't spoken about it much; else when we have he's said 'you've got Helen, I've got John'. But it's not the same.

Being deaf and dumb, I think Mr Holt missed this exchange: he did not want to make a comment himself. The others who had no children were at pains to point out that they were in some way different, and their marriage was strong enough without children.

> Not in the sense that they would save a marriage. I'm heartily glad we never had any as things turned out. I don't think that was the deciding factor. I would like to get married again, but I wouldn't say that I'd want to be assured that she could have children before getting married. But if I do I'd certainly be keen to have children. (Mr Carter)

> Staying together and helping one another comes higher on the list than children. (Mr Turner)

Most of those asserting that children are very important were parents.

> It's selfish if people get married and can have children, but don't have them, because reason for marriage is having children.   (Mr Carver)

Mrs Carver, however, did not agree with her husband.

A fairly representative view of those who had children was given by the Quicks.

> Never really felt married until we had children. The mundane things are worth it.   (Mr Quick)

> In some ways 'yes', but not all. You shouldn't have a baby to save a marriage or it will end up on the rocks. But in a happy marriage it makes you work at it – gives you a sense of purpose. It completes your marriage – it's something very special, but they won't save a marriage.   (Mrs Quick)

The pronatalist assumptions about the indivisibility of marriage and children referred to in Chapter 3 are still evident amongst some of these couples, but the general emphasis was on children being just one important element, with the key being the quality of the marital relationship itself.

REMAINING CHILDLESS

Eight (27 per cent) couples withdrew from investigation and treatment before the point at which the Clinic reported that no more could be done for them. Two significant associations emerged in relation to these couples. Firstly, of the eight withdrawing, only one woman was occupationally defined as 'working class' (i.e. Registrar General IIIM, IV, V). This suggested an under-representation significant beyond the 1 per cent level (χ^2 =7.912, $P<0.01$). There was no similar significance for the men. This is surprising; it might have been expected that the working-class women, who are likely to be less articulate, might more readily drop out of such a demanding procedure. The reverse was the case. This might be due to the deference factor discussed by Cartwright and Anderson (1981) in seeking to explain the lower rate of complaints from their working-class patients. With such small numbers, this must be regarded as an issue of interest, not a firm prediction.

Secondly, it was found that all those who withdrew were rated as having close contact with their family (that is, at least weekly visits if living near by or contact by other means if living at a distance) (χ^2=5.185, $P<0.025$); contact with friends was not significantly different. Abandoning the quest for children might be said to be a particularly difficult period, involving a final acceptance that pregnancy is very unlikely, and the recognition that continuing might have borne fruit, albeit at considerable, personal sacrifice. In such a situation the support of family might be especially important.

> Carry on as we are; never considered anything else . . . All family and close friends know; we're not the type of people to hide things; we just tell people. Initially we was upset, but resigned to it now, if it's not to be. They think about what will happen if anything happens to Dan; but it doesn't do to think too far ahead. When people ask I just say we can't have any. That's usually the end of it.   (Mrs Underwood)

Incidentally, Mrs Underwood was the only respondent to mention surrogacy. This became 'headline news' with the Baby Cotton case, in which custody was given in favour of the 'contracting' parents in January 1985. This judgement was followed swiftly by the banning of agency surrogacy in the United Kingdom by the Surrogacy Arrangements Act 1985. The majority of the final interviews were conducted during this period; yet no other couple mentioned the issue.

> Surrogate is taking things too far. I think it's profiteering paying £6,500 for a baby; what if she changes her mind? It's all a bit distasteful.
>   (Mrs Underwood)

The hypothesised association between male infertility and early withdrawal from treatment did not emerge. Of the eight withdrawals, in three cases there was a male deficit, in four cases it was a female deficit, and in one the deficit was shared. The only two female respondents approached to take part in the study who subsequently declined, did so because the husband refused; in both cases a male problem was diagnosed and they withdrew at an early stage of the process. To this extent, there might be more substance to the hypothesis than the study itself showed.

Both of the couples who were not fully interviewed remained childless. The Greens will be considered in relation to adoption and fostering. Mrs Green was unwilling to be interviewed at the final contact. After considerable investigation, problems had been found with both of them. Little could be offered for his poor semen quality beyond DI; for Mrs Green there was the possibility of hormonal treatment for an asynchronous cycle and a laparotomy to deal with adhesions. They were on the waiting list for both procedures when they decided to withdraw.

Mrs Carter continued in treatment for anovulation although she and her husband separated quite early on, without her establishing another relationship. She declined to be interviewed after the first time, although promising interviews to me on the telephone several times.

In only one case, the Truswells, was the withdrawal a clearly decided event. In all others the couple appeared to have drifted to a decision as the chances of achieving a pregnancy appeared to recede. The Kitchens mentioned that two-and-a-half years' investigation was long enough for them, they would 'let nature take its course'. The Youngs spoke of missing an appointment, because Mrs Young was anxious what the result might be. Despite wanting to know the results, they never overcame their reluctance to face the Clinic staff again. The appointments system in the Clinic was such that couples who were as tentative or ambivalent as the Youngs might slip through unnoticed. If an appointment was missed, only occasionally would another appointment be made; normally it was left to the initiative of the couple to request a further time.

The Dorairajes noted the increased ambivalence felt towards pregnancy by those who had become adjusted to a lifestyle without children.

> If we did have a child now, it would be a bit of a problem. We could adjust, but we're rooted in our social life now . . . you gradually adjust to a different way of life. (Mr Dorairaj)

The *Truswells* were the only couple who, having found the extent of their problems, made a positive decision to end the uncertainty, and thus made a positive statement of being *childfree*.

The Truswells were high educational achievers; he to degree level and she to 'A' levels. Mr Truswell was an industrial engineer, his wife an office supervisor, with the same large industrial concern. During the study period they moved with their employers out of the area. They had a high standard of living, and a comfortable home. They were apparently an outgoing couple who talked equally and freely of their situation.

No abnormality was detected in Mrs Truswell's case; she had a satisfactory HSG but refused to undergo laparoscopy:

> We don't want to rush into all the investigations . . . I was amazed they came back to me; felt they were clutching at straws. (Mrs Truswell)

She had a termination of pregnancy seven years previously at nine weeks' gestation, and expected not to have major problems.

Mr Truswell was diagnosed as suffering a maturation defect of spermatogenesis which might respond to treatment. The diagnostic testicular biopsy was very painful, and they withdrew at this point, although very satisfied with the way this problem had been handled, without pursuing the possibility of hormonal treatment.

They found it difficult to discuss their problems with each other, although not, it seemed, with me. Both had talked to close friends without telling the other, and admitted to long periods of not mentioning it. Both volunteered that an outsider (myself) facilitated the discussion they needed but could not initiate on their own. They were one of only two couples to feel that the process went too quickly; particularly thinking they would have been glad for the initial appointment to have been delayed. He had some warning of the oligospermia as he had assessed his own semen whilst a biochemistry student, but this did not prevent Mr Truswell experiencing the diagnosis as a personal blow, commenting

> It's been hard; like living under a cloud, dinted my self-confidence. If it had been out of the blue, don't know how I would have coped. For the first couple of months I felt 'why me?' 'Why can everyone else do it and not me?' Infertility still has a stigma of being unmanly.

After nearly nine months' investigation they thought it unlikely they would consider adopting, but recognised they might feel different in a couple of years 'after we're 30'.

> Not prepared to go through long periods of chemical treatment or operations and still be uncertain of having children. We don't see ourselves going for another nine months. . . Currently we don't want children anyway because of new commitments [i.e. job].
>
> (Mr Truswell)

When they were seen for the last time, they had moved with promotion to jobs a hundred miles away. They had passed the, for them, significant ages of 30 and firmly decided to have no children.

> Neither of us wanted to start a late family. We were told you've only got one-in-a-thousand chance, and would have wanted two, so it could be one-in-a-million. It wouldn't be what we wanted.   (Mr Truswell)

> We were offered more tests on me, given men with lower sperm counts have had children . . . couldn't be bothered. Your life's half over if you're not careful. We were settled into our own life – we'd changed round totally.   (Mrs Truswell)

They decided that Mr Truswell should have a vasectomy.

> Did not bother me; just removing the one-in-a-thousand chance . . . Didn't want you to go back on the pill at that age [i.e. 30].
>
> (Mr Truswell)

> It was more annoying to have to convince the GP.   (Mrs Truswell)

> Once I'd got over the hurdle of accepting the low sperm count, there was no other hurdle to get over . . . putting wife back on the pill would be stupid – no, irresponsible. Seemed easiest thing.   (Mr Truswell)

They had many criticisms of the Infertility Clinic, but in summary:

> If anyone was desperate to have children, I'd still recommend they go [there]; but they'd need to be desperate. Perhaps we were never desperate enough.
>
> (Mr Truswell)

Adoption had been discussed, but they claimed that DI never crossed their minds.

> In the event I remember saying that if I couldn't have our own, I didn't want anyone else's.
>
> (Mrs Truswell)

The picture they painted was of a close relationship:

> A bit closer than other couples who've just decided not to have children. We've been through quite a lot together. Hard to know; don't know if we are closer, or just that we feel we ought to be. Don't know how close we'd be anyway.
>
> (Mrs Truswell)

> Maybe brought us closer . . . we got married for life.   (Mr Truswell)

> We'd rather go out together than separately. We don't need time out on our own. We know there'll only ever be the two of us; there'll be no scapegoats; we have to sort it out.
>
> (Mrs Truswell)

Although they saw children as important, they did not see them as essential to a secure marriage.

> We're a strong couple; don't need an anchor to hang onto.
>
> (Mr Truswell)

> Not us! We don't need kids to keep us together.   (Mrs Truswell)

The Truswells seemed a confident and relaxed couple, who related easily. Mrs Truswell was the more edgy and nervous of the two. It was clear that talking about feelings was very unusual for them, several times things were admitted which surprised the other. The final interview was a very long one, which they openly said was a helpful opportunity to talk about things in a way they usually avoided. The move of home and jobs was just part of a clear decision to set out on a new course in life, which would not include the possibility of children, and look to the advantages that this offered without dwelling on the things they would miss. The Truswells were the clearest example in this study of the 'voluntarily' childless couple for whom being without children is a case of making a virtue of necessity.

Investigation and treatment for infertility will only help some of those who embark on the course. As indicated, as many as half of those will remain childless. Those who do not succeed will need to find alternative sources of satisfaction and means of identification for the relationship; for some the alternative will not include children.

DONOR INSEMINATION: DI

Note: At the time of these interviews, the term 'artificial insemination by donor' (AID) was still the accepted usage. As one of the respondents noted, this acronym has become unacceptable for the confusion raised with acquired immune deficiency syndrome (AIDS), which is now such a widely discussed concern. I have adopted the course of referring throughout to DI to avoid this confusion, although the reader must remember that the medical services and patients all used the term AID at the time of the study.

For those couples where the principal component in their reduced fertility is a deficit in the man's sperm quality, DI is an available route to parenthood. This provides what Snowden *et al.* (1983) term 'nurturing' parenthood for the father and 'complete' parenthood for the mother.

DI seems to have been practised since the end of the eighteenth century in this country, but only in very recent years has it become a matter for public discussion. Although mechanically simple, as far as is known the procedure has always been the responsibility of doctors. Some feminists have begun to argue strongly for the resources and techniques to be widely available in order to facilitate women choosing their own path to fertility, free of what is perceived to be male/medical hegemony (cf. Arditti and Duelli Klein 1984). As well as being part of a wider feminist claim for women to exert control over their own bodies and their potential for motherhood, this may in part be a response to the widespread hostility amongst the medical profession to the insemination of lesbian and unmarried women (e.g. Foss 1982). Allied to IVF, DI provides the possibility of so-called virgin births which aroused a storm of popular controversy when given publicity in the UK press in 1991.

DI has always been regarded as a remedy for childlessness that should be kept as secret as possible; even the child has not been informed of its origins, let alone family and wider society. A thorough discussion of the ethical and moral issues surrounding DI is available in *Artificial Reproduction* by Snowden *et al.* (1983). The moral position remains confused. Both Judaism and Roman Catholicism consider DI to be adultery. A commission established by the Archbishop of Canterbury (1948) condemned the practice of DI as immoral and wished it to become a criminal offence. The Feversham Committee (1960) was the last official report to condemn DI as socially undesirable. Since that time there has been a steadily growing public awareness and acceptance of the procedure and discussion of its implications. It is now accepted by most non-Catholic, Christian denominations.

The legal position has now been clarified. It is estimated that some 2,000 DI births are now achieved annually in the UK: an accurate figure cannot yet be given as the requirement of official notification was only implemented with the Human Fertilisation and Embryology Act 1990. The Family Law Reform Act 1987 determined that the offspring of DI undertaken with the consent of both marital partners should be regarded legally as the legitimate offspring of the marriage, in line with the recommendations of the Warnock Report (1984). All the previous studies (Snowden and Mitchell 1981, Foss 1982, Owens 1983, Snowden *et al.* 1983) record all DI parents appearing to take the course this and all other services seemed to assume (if not actively advise) – 'register him/her as your own': the position now sanctioned by law.

The secrecy surrounding the procedure is still very intense. Snowden *et al.* helpfully stress the need to distinguish 'secrecy', 'confidentiality' and 'anonymity'. The tendency at the time in DI services was to encourage secrecy, whereby no one, the child included, should be told any details of origin, and the child is presented to the world as a natural child of the marriage. If confidentiality were the main principle, parents would still have the right to share knowledge with those they wish to know, including the child, whilst remaining certain that medical confidentiality will not be compromised; the initiative remains with the parents and they could be encouraged to share the knowledge with the child, as is now strongly advocated in adoption. Anonymity could still be guaranteed to the donor, which would not prevent general details of social and medical background being shared, whilst protecting the donor from legal suits of paternity. Owens' survey for NAC, and NAC's lobby document to MPs during the debate on the Human Fertilisation and Embryology Bill, confirmed the strong support for secrecy amongst childless couples, particularly those who had resolved their childlessness via DI. The trend, exemplified by the proposals (Department of Health 1990) for more open adoption arrangements, permitting continuing contact between birth and adoptive parents, is, however, in the opposite direction. The Human Fertilisation and Embryology Act and the associated Code of Practice will, in the future, provide for those born as a result of DI to have information about their genetic parentage after counselling. Secrecy will not be entirely possible. The conservative approach was adopted amongst the couples in this study.

Two different clinical services operated during the time of this study. In the first year or so couples wishing to consider DI, after an initial discussion with the doctor in the Infertility Clinic, were referred to a consultant in chemical pathology, who offered DI both privately and on the NHS. The latter involved up to 18 months' waiting, and was strictly limited to one course of eight cycles, two inseminations per cycle. The only difference between the NHS and private services was the wait for the first insemination and the number of inseminations given. This doctor gave the couple an advisory interview which explained the technicalities of the procedure and some of the legal issues. They were then usually seen by a trained marriage guidance counsellor who would help the couple to explore the emotional aspects and implications of DI. Insemination would be performed if no serious problems emerged. Three respondent couples were seen under this system, two on the NHS.

Thereafter the Infertility Clinic instituted a private service (in the same sense as the IVF service (i.e. fees paid were below full cost and contributed to the funds supporting the work of the University Department)). This was designed to conform more closely to their own practices in relation to ovulation monitoring and general management. In this service the responsible woman doctor was also a trained family planning counsellor who provided both medical advice and counselling. Three couples used this service. It should be noted that comments from couples in the study refer to both services.

DI offers the possibility of 'complete' parenthood to the wife in the phrase of Snowden *et al.* (1983) – that is, she provides the ovum, and thus half the genetic material, as in normal conception; she then carries the child to birth and subsequently nurtures that child. Although the husband does not provide the sperm, nor, therefore, any genetic contribution, he will become the nurturing or social parent for the child. Unlike adoption, therefore, the child is genetically half the child of the marriage, and in all other respects can be treated as a natural child of the marriage. At the time of this study, because there is a pregnancy and the cloak of secrecy is available to shroud the circumstances of conception, it was perfectly possible for couples to deny to anyone, including the child, the nature of the child's parentage.

The expectation of secrecy assumed that DI services took trouble to match donors to 'parents' for blood group, colouring, stature, etc., as did that operated in association with the Infertility Clinic. In practice it seems that many DI services do not take this trouble. In Owens' (1983) and Snowden *et al.*'s (1983) research the dissimilarity of hair or eye colour had often been the trigger for DI parents to reveal to the growing child the details of conception. Foss (1982) reports using just 25 donors to achieve 308 pregnancies in 381 women, which precludes careful matching. Recent developments in genetic 'fingerprinting' would make even the most careful matching inadequate, but it could still enable public deception. These developments were powerful arguments for a change in the attitudes to secrecy, which now see practice moving in the direction of considerable openness taken by adoption. The consultant argued for encouraging openness about DI, particularly with the child. There was no evidence that the couples interviewed heard or heeded this view.

As has been seen, DI was not considered an option by many of these couples early in their treatment. With the diagnosis of male subfertility more were encouraged to consider it. Of the 13 couples for whom it would have been appropriate to consider DI, 11 (37 per cent of the total group) had indeed thought of this alternative but five had rejected it, whilst six pursued it – three to conception and birth during the course of the study. The first clinic quoted a conception rate of 60 per cent of women treated, Foss (1982) 68 per cent, Snowden *et al.* (1983) 76.7 per cent. One husband for whom DI did not succeed commented wryly that it only cost £3 a time for his cattle and worked every time. In no clinic does it 'work every time' for people.

The main factor mentioned for considering it seriously was the 'genetic' argument used by the Carvers who successfully had a DI child:

> Plumped for DI as the wife was keen to experience birth and a baby would be 50 per cent our own which is better than 0 per cent. Would not have ruled it out. (Mr Carver)

Those who rejected the idea mostly confined their comments to 'just don't like the idea' (Mrs Underwood). Blizzard's book (1977) has already been cited for its moving account of the pains of male sterility and the threat to his self-esteem which DI can represent to the husband. Crowe (1987) noted male resistance to IVF/DI because of the importance to men of the genetic link in fatherhood. One woman did make plain the concern that it might be seen by the husband as a further assault on his masculinity:

> I was very upset at the suggestion. I didn't tell Manny, I know he'd be very upset at the idea; he wouldn't like it. (Mrs Holt)

The extent of confiding was very limited amongst those who went ahead. Two told no one at all, two only told the wife's mother/parents and two also included the husband's parents and close friends. Half of the couples studied by Amuzu *et al.* (1990) told no one.

The Mitchells confided in the wife's family (N.B. not his), but they subsequently firmly maintained, untruthfully, to everyone (including the GP and me) that they conceived naturally, soon after withdrawing from DI. The Clinic doctor was in no doubt that this conception was indeed DI; it therefore seemed that this couple had changed their minds about disclosing the information, and were prepared to go to some trouble to 'cover their tracks'. The same ability to deny an uncomfortable situation has already been discussed at some length in relation to Mr Mitchell's semen analysis (p. 105 above). The frailty of the position they chose to adopt suggested that, in their case, the counselling which they had received had not enabled them to work through all their feelings about his subfertility and DI before she became pregnant.

The two couples to discuss the idea fairly widely, at least in principle, both knew personally someone else who had undergone DI, unlike the other couples. On the whole they reported supportive attitudes from the people they told, with one exception:

> They [family] think it's great; mother thinks it's great. One friend doesn't believe in it, but that's a load of old rubbish – she's got a child, they should think what it feels like. If you've got a couple really wanting a baby, people don't understand because they've got a baby. Mind you, I'm not sure how I'd feel if someone else said 'she's had a baby but it's not Graham's'.   (Mrs Grindrod)

Those who talked to their parents reported positive responses, although some initial hesitancy in one case. Mrs Carver's mother paid the DI fees. There was a noticeable reluctance amongst all these couples to tell the husband's parents.

One of those who had a child through DI suffered post-natal depression. This was treated by her GP with supportive counselling and short-term medication, and quickly resolved. They were both adamant that the circumstances of the birth had not caused the depression:

> I never felt bad towards Irene. Life was wonderful for the first few months, then it happened . . . I never thought about where she came from; just a matter of hormones; also all the worries about the house and no extra money coming in . . . Doctor took account of it all; mainly talk – pleased that they dealt with it in that way.   (Mrs Carver)

The impact of DI has been exceptionally hard to study because of the surrounding secrecy. Several follow-up studies have been conducted; however, only the most recent of them has been able to collect detailed information on this topic (Amuzu *et al.* 1990). It has been possible to identify the number of marriages which failed up to the point of follow-up; although all studies are open to two criticisms: the high rate of non-responders could well conceal those worst affected; follow-up periods are sometimes very short (e.g. Foss 1982). Stanway, with an unquoted source, suggests that an American study found only one subsequent divorce amongst 800 couples who applied for DI; and that couple had been turned down.

Couples who have a DI baby have far more stable marriages than those who have children normally.

(Stanway 1984: 183)

He ascribes this to the trials of infertility; the stresses which precede the decision to seek DI; the investment of the husband in 'making up for his fault'. He declares, with little evidence:

For the man social fatherhood is more important than genetic fatherhood.

(Stanway 1984: 185)

Snowden *et al.* (1983) report 0.3 per cent couples abandoning DI because of marital disharmony. Foss (1982) notes one known divorce in 564 couples seen. The Humphreys (1987) found two couples in 100 divorcing. Amuzu *et al.* (1990) confirmed this situation, having studied 427 women treated over a 12-year period, with only 7.2 per cent subsequently divorcing, well below the population norm. The view is strongly presented in the literature that, once a decision is made to pursue the option of DI, the marriages are remarkably resilient. There was no reason to disbelieve this view on the basis of this study.

Four of the six couples proceeding found the doctor and counsellor helpful. However, as one of the pathologist's patients only saw the doctor, and the Infertility Clinic's own service only involved the doctor, this left only two of the couples who had an opportunity of separate counselling. On the whole the response was positive, although one saw it as:

Shock treatment; no comeback on them if anything went wrong. We were fairly determined from the word go: couldn't have been side-tracked by them.

(Mr Turner)

Can't remember them very well; you see that many people. Had talked about it ourselves, so made no difference.

(Mrs Turner)

We don't think we need help from anyone; they are there to do what they're paid for. It's a marvellous service for such as us – but it didn't work.

(Mr Turner)

Only one couple felt they did not have enough help in deciding about DI; but four of the couples felt that it was their own decision, and no one else could have helped very much.

The principal concern expressed by these couples was over the issue of confidentiality, or 'secrecy' as Snowden *et al.* (1983) would define it.

Feel as if the whole world knows after being told it was so secret . . . You wonder how many people get to read the notes.

(Mrs Carver)

A specific concern was raised by this couple which suggests that the pathology service operated in ways that may not take sufficient account of the feelings of their patients. Perhaps partly because of the logistical problems created by using fresh rather than frozen semen, matching seemed not to be attempted and no provision was made for subsequent children.

Got a shock when we went to ask about number 2. There isn't one! Told it isn't possible to use the same donor.   (Mr Carver)

Nice to think there would be some resemblance . . . We've already had comments about it; Irene not looking like him. If this one is very different again, it will increase the questioning.   (Mrs Carver)

The other source of criticism, which seemed to be directed at the first service only, was the practical and emotional context: one couple were very unhappy at the DI being given during a regular clinic; another described the process itself as 'degrading', 'horrid' and 'impersonal'. One couple receiving the second service, however, described it as much more caring:

We had the same Sister; she was very kind; we felt she cared very much, and it was very private.   (Mrs Mitchell)

The experience of the three couples attending the first clinic strongly supported the view of Snowden *et al.* (1983) and the Warnock Report (1984) that some general standards should be set to control the operation of DI services, which will now be assured by the Human Fertilisation and Embryology Authority established by the 1990 Act.

Not surprisingly most of the satisfaction noted with DI involved the three who achieved a pregnancy.

None of the couples intended to tell the child the facts of its paternity. They all intended to 'shut it out of our memory' (Mr Turner), and denied that it would make any difference to their feelings towards the child.

The experience and feelings of the *Trevors* helpfully illustrate typical reactions to the *DI route to parenthood*. The Trevors were a quiet couple, very upset at their failure to conceive a child. Mr Trevor took the lead in the interviews, but took pains to check out his views with his wife. They were both skilled manual workers, not previously married. They owned their comfortable home.

After two semen analyses and a testicular biopsy, Mr Trevor was diagnosed as being severely oligospermic, having no motile (i.e. forward moving) sperm, an increased number of abnormal forms and decreased count. This was found to be a case of severe early maturation arrest, insusceptible to treatment. Mrs Trevor was found to have no abnormality, being assessed to the stage of HSG. The Trevors had told no one about their being investigated for infertility apart from her mother. They were very anxious for reassurance about the confidentiality of their participation in the research, particularly at the final interview when their child had been born.

The Trevors were one of those couples to feel strongly about the manner in which they were given the news about his subfertility.

> When he told him, all the nurses and student doctors were in; it weren't private enough.   (Mrs Trevor)

Mr Trevor admitted the impact the diagnosis had on his self-image.

> I felt a he-man at school; it made me feel less of a man.

He also made the point many more men must now feel in the wake of recent publicity that:

> To start with it felt degrading . . . They need to change the name with that disease [i.e. AIDS] going round.

They were concerned for the privacy of the actual insemination, and the problem of getting time off work each month for the insemination appointment. Even the treatment rooms used were felt inadequate in this regard: these were curtained off out-patient cubicles, not the separate consulting rooms used in the second service.

They reported enjoying talking to the counsellor about DI, and found it helpful to put their trust in her, although this was not without ambivalence.

> Said she wanted us to be genuine. She sat and listened. She did it well.
> (Mr Trevor)

> That's her job. Wonder why you have to see her? After a couple's been married so long, surely they must be stable enough to have children. Seems like they're prying a bit. It was us own decision.   (Mrs Trevor)

The Trevors decided to put the whole experience behind them, and, despite the diagnosis given him, Mr Trevor could still argue:

> We still don't know if he's mine or the hospital's. We're convinced he's mine; what he looked like at birth, time of the month and so on.

Both agreed that whilst not essential to a marriage 'it's not complete without children'. Perhaps not coincidentally this final interview was one of the shortest conducted; the concern to put DI out of their minds was very apparent and, although they were entirely co-operative, my interview was an unwelcome reminder.

As with other changes in the organisation of the Infertility Clinic, it appeared that the change of approach experienced by some of the couples had been an improvement on the original service. Further attention to the concerns being expressed could see further improvement. The attitudes of these couples to the concealment of DI were typical of those reported in the literature. There was no evidence here to contradict the optimistic views of other research that DI does not of itself constitute a threat to the stability of marriage.

ADOPTION AND FOSTERING

None of these couples had previously applied to foster or adopt. Not surprisingly, when asked about alternatives in the early months of the investigation, adoption was the most considered, if unsuccessful in having their own child. The misleading advice of some GPs, as discussed already, could be a factor in encouraging couples to hope for what has become a very scarce opportunity.

Most couples seemed to be aware that adoption is not an easily obtained option, notwithstanding the doctors who seem to believe that it can be 'prescribed'. There were substantial misgivings even at the early stage. Several couples already felt they would not wish to consider parenting another person's child:

> Couldn't adopt, not the same: couldn't love it like me own.
>
> (Mrs Flower)

Part of the uncertainty was the well-known requirement of social work vetting:

> I objected to the implication that 'we will decide whether you are fit parents'. Ordinary folk don't get investigated.   (Mr Keith)

By the final visit, 16 (53 per cent) couples had at some time in the process considered the possibility of adoption; four had dismissed the idea, as they felt unable to accept another's child. Six couples had actually applied to an adoption agency: one had been turned down; one had been accepted; one started going to preparatory meetings; but three had not even begun the process. These last four had all been warned that there would be a sub-stantial delay, possibly of years, before the application could be assessed, let alone a child placed.

One of the couples, the Youngs, had been accepted to adopt and a baby placed – this was much more quickly than usual, given the extreme shortage of babies for adoption. They had applied in April 1983 and a child was placed in June 1984 – almost unheard of speed in recent years for a 'normal, healthy, white baby'. They spoke very warmly of the help they received from the social workers who had vetted their application and placed the child. At the final interview they were anticipating with concern the hearing of the adoption order which was to be contested by the natural mother, who had revoked her consent. They felt Mark, their baby, was 'just like us own', and were understandably anxious about the outcome.

The possibility of losing a child placed for adoption made the Underwoods decide not to consider either adoption or fostering. The social work literature concerning the recruitment of substitute families emphasises the importance of clarifying motivation: in the case of childless couples, the concern is expressed that they might seek to foster in the unrealistic expectation that this is a short cut to adoption, for which they would have applied had it been possible (Rowe 1969, DHSS 1976, Aldgate 1982). However, there seemed to be no confusion amongst these couples about the essential differences between adoption and fostering. Most said they would not consider fostering because of its essentially temporary nature.

Equally, the matter of their own ages was often mentioned. All of the couples considering adoption who were approaching (or had passed) 30 expressed anxiety that their age might make it impossible. Several commented bitterly on the injustice, as they saw it, of age limits. This exacerbated complaints about the length of time taken in the investigations.

> I'd rather go for DI than adoption. Don't agree with those rules about ages. I'm always looking after other people's children . . . What can I do, if you could tell me . . . . what can I do if adoption societies won't entertain me? Fostering? [*her own suggestion*] that I couldn't do . . . I'd never want them to go back. No, couldn't do that.   (Mrs Grindrod)

Amongst those who had seriously considered adoption, it was striking that most had discussed it with family and often friends. They all seemed to have received support for the idea.

> Most people are supportive; parents totally keen. Quite a few friends of mine know people or had friends who had been adopted, and they all said 'great'. I never heard one negative comment . . . couldn't see who would ever be suitable if we weren't.   (Mr Mitchell)

This couple, who have been discussed in relation to DI, made the revealing comment that they were going to withdraw from the adoption application as they 'got more and more worried about the telling part of it'. They had started adoption preparation groups which had been emphasising the importance of telling the child of its adoptive status from the beginning. They decided not to 'tell' anyone at all, their GP included, about DI.

The two couples who had spoken to 'no one, only you' were also the only two who had only a male problem. They, also, were not willing to consider DI.

The situation of the *Greens* who had been *rejected for adoption* is of interest in this connection, although their story is far from typical. This couple avoided contact for the final interview for some time, and when an appointment was finally made, Mrs Green went out at the agreed time to avoid the interview. Her husband explained apologetically that she had been so upset by their disappointments over infertility investigation and adoption that she did not wish to be interviewed. They had hoped to adopt, and had fostered for some time.

The Greens had both been married before, and had been in this relationship for almost six years when referred to the Infertility Clinic, although married for just two years. Both worked, she as a shop assistant and he as a care assistant. They lived in a flat on a large council estate. Mr Green had been unable to have children with his first wife over a period of four years, but had not been investigated; Mrs Green had not attempted to have children in the first marriage.

The investigations showed that he had severe oligospermia, caused by arrested maturity which could not be treated. Mrs Green was shown to have one tube blocked, ovarian cysts and fine adhesions. At first contact they impressed as a close couple, in which Mr Green took the lead, being very talkative and articulate. Neither seemed quick to understand complicated matters, and instructions about questionnaires required careful, repeated explanation. His wife was much the quieter and seemed the more anxious. Both said that it was she who had been most upset by their failure to have children.

The Greens had applied to adopt before attending the Infertility Clinic. They had been summarily rejected on the grounds that they had not undergone investigation, and had not been legally married for two years, although they had co-habited for four years prior to their marriage a year previously. They were very angry at what seemed to them a peremptory dismissal. However, they had also been befriending a child in residential care and were being vetted as foster parents.

They always attended the Clinic together, and were generally positive about the service, although critical of the time it all took, the lack of explanations and the changing doctors in particular. Like other couples where the husband had a clearly identified problem, they were confused by the focus on Mrs Green.

> It's my problem, but they've done more for her than me. I should have been in hospital; feel very disappointed sometimes.   (Mr Green)

The Clinic failed to explain the reasons for investigating the woman thoroughly where a problem had already been identified on the man's side. Clinic practice was subsequently fully vindicated in this case in view of the diagnosis of her problems. For a period, the failure to explain this practice exacerbated their irritation with the lack of explanation, and meant that they felt distanced from the process.

> I was annoyed at them, getting ratty and not explaining what the jargon meant – despite persisting, they wouldn't explain properly.
>
> (Mr Green)

As with several of the women, Mrs Green, when she was admitted for the laparoscopy, felt the doctors on the ward took more trouble to explain carefully what was being done, and the meaning of the results obtained. (The doctors, although unrecognised, were often the same people, although reactions suggested that they had more time to explain results properly than in the Clinic.) She was one, also, to be upset by her fellow in-patients' situations; she shared a ward with four women, all being sterilised.

Mr Green described the emotional impact of their investigation graphically:

> Feels like a corridor of doors, each shutting in front of you. One knock after another . . . bit of a slaughter house all the way round.

They both said that 'it helps to talk to people like you', but felt it difficult to confide in friends and family as they would like. However, this feeling was to change for her by the final follow-up four-and-a-half years after first attending the Clinic. Mrs Green then refused to be interviewed although I was able to have a general discussion with her husband. His account of the intervening years was a moving one, worth recounting at length; it is repeated here just as it was recorded:

> After we gave up with Sheffield [Clinic] we took to fostering. We had 24 children over 2 years, up to five at a time, old and young. We really threw ourselves into it. I think if I'm honest now it was me on an ego trip. We'd do better than anyone else. What gets me now – I feel a real hypocrite. I was teaching foster parents, you know, that Parenting Plus [*teaching package for foster parents*]. I'd tell 'em, 'see all, hear all, say nowt' – but I never saw all or heard all; I did say nowt though! It leaves you feeling bitter, you don't want to, but you do.
>
> [*Applied to foster, approved; specifically wanted children with a view to adoption. Then applied to adopt, turned down.*]
>
> It was a conflict of personalities really; I didn't get on with the adoptions woman. I disagreed with her in front of a meeting. I said 'How can you sit in judgement when you've never had any children?' That didn't go down very well. She was an older woman – she's moved on now, retired that is. A bit Victorian in her ideas about children and

parents. We were offered the chance to appeal, decided not; we'd continue fostering.

We had a pair of kids for a year, girl was 11 and the boy 6; mother is alcoholic. The social worker intended long term with a view to adoption; the senior social worker wanted to give the mother another chance. She'd never done anything to earn it – never stopped drinking. She had the kids home, it lasted 6 weeks – they lived on biscuits. The social worker asked us to have them back. The wife didn't want to, but I said 'let's give it a try for the kids' sake'. This was a year ago; it lasted a week and Else walked out. She just rang up she was going – left the kids and me. Social workers said she'd technically abandoned them. I tried to cope but they wouldn't have let me, being a man on my own, the girl being 11. The wife soon came back.

We never talk about kids now. Don't get me wrong, we have friends with little ones, she'll pick them up and give them a love. But she says it's nice to hand them back. I think the spark's gone – that feeling for wanting children. Maybe it'll change . . . She won't talk about it – feels very bitter about social workers an' that. She let them know she was finding it hard, but they didn't listen. Mind you I didn't either.

The woman bears the strain. I was out at work. Then, many of the kids, they had been living with their mother, they were happy with me as father for the time being. But they had a mother, didn't want Else. That little girl could be very spiteful, tell tales, that sort of thing. I thought we'd manage. Wanted to be real good at fostering – get on with things, not bother the social worker, sort ourselves out. That sort of thing. That's why I did the teaching. You have to have a motive – be a bit selfish if you like. I never believed these couples who said they wanted to help just; give a child a home. You've got to want to get something out of it. We wanted children of us own, that was bottom of it.

Nobody ever wanted me; I spent 15 years in [*children's*] homes, but they clung on to you then, and there weren't all the foster parents or adopters then there are now.

But it left her so she didn't want to think about it. I know what's more important to me. Don't get me wrong, I'd like children, but the marriage is more important. But there's not much chance now – unless we suddenly get lots of money. But I still fire blanks [infertile semen], so test tube [*IVF*] wouldn't work.

[*Re. wife's 'breakdown'*] I should have seen it coming. Wife has it all to do in fostering. She'd go to bed by 9 – but she'd get up cheery in the morning, so I thought she was alright. Then she just cracked. Rang me at work to say she was going. Came back a few days later; but that was it as far as Social Services were concerned. Now she doesn't even want to think about it; we don't talk about it.

I hope you see now – perhaps you can piece it together. It's all related; getting turned down by Clinic, the fostering, then being turned down for adoption. Like the doctor said 'perhaps it wasn't meant to be'.

Mr Green expresses clearly the way that childless people are seen by social services, just as in the literature reviewed in Chapter 1; they constitute a resource. The hard-pressed child care agency easily neglects the profound truth Mr Green puts his finger on, that motivation is crucial. The pressures under which social work agencies find themselves can lead to gross abuse of substitute parents; adoption is jealously guarded as demand exceeds supply, but in fostering, where the reverse obtains, the childless couple can be used beyond their capabilities.

There is no suggestion that the Greens are typical of the experience of childless couples who seek to foster or adopt, or that they did not present considerable problems for any assessing social worker. They do highlight some very important issues concerning the way these services operate, and the help that is available to childless people in making up their own minds about how they should deal with the frustration of their primary wish – a child of their own.

As long as 'normal, healthy, white children' are in short supply for adoption, some childless couples are going to be attracted, or inveigled, into fostering, which will not meet their needs. The key must be a readily available social work service, liaising closely with the infertility service, which helps them to identify their own needs, and come to terms with the reality of what is available.

The couples interviewed demonstrated an accurate understanding of the crucial difference between adoption, permanent substitute parenthood, and fostering, temporarily acting on behalf of a local authority *in loco parentis* for a child needing care away from the natural family. It was only too well appreciated that, in present circumstances, it is very difficult to find an agency willing to accept a couple for adoption; and that this is a very long process. The age restrictions were one of the sources of unease generated by the period taken by hospital investigation. The requirement in adoption that couples had to be assessed by social workers was known and understood, although generally disliked. In summary, these interviews showed that childless couples are aware of the many constraints which surround the adoption service, and the general nature of modern child placement practice.

CHILDREN

This is the outcome probably all of the patients at an Infertility Clinic are looking for when they are referred. This is not to say that all want children, with equal single-mindedness, at any cost, or that their importance does not change. As has been noted already, the Clinic could perhaps have done more to negotiate the extent to which each couple wanted to pursue this goal.

Sixteen (53 per cent) of the couples did have a child after investigation at the Clinic, five of these without active treatment. All of these children were healthy, full-term babies who were thriving when seen at the final interview. (The Monks had only just conceived at this time.) The nature of the problem that was identified in each case can be seen recorded in Tables 4.2 and 4.3.

The importance of their emotional state was also mentioned by these couples in 'explaining' how they came to conceive.

> Just got a job: that's why I fell. (Mrs Ivy)

> I still think it was partly stopping worrying about a baby when your grandmother died, and you were worrying about your mother; that's when you actually fell. (Mr Mitchell)

> I think that week-end in the Lake District did it; had a marvellous week-end, really relaxed, smashing. (Mrs Mitchell)

It has already been noted that having a child enabled these couples to restate the importance of children to a marriage more strongly than those who had not been successful.

Although no attempt was made to 'measure' the involvement of these parents with their child, a clear impression was given by some that confirmed the whispered comment of the midwife to one mother 'he'll be a really special baby!'

> Children are very precious when you've waited for them. You have to be very careful or you'd end up with a spoiled little brat. (Mr Flower)

Four of the mothers mentioned not being willing to leave their child with anyone else for any length of time:

> We won't leave her, no one baby-sits her locally . . . have to consider her in everything we do. (Mrs Coleman)

The different situation of Mrs Butler has already been mentioned in this regard; from her baby's birth she returned to full-time work and employed a nanny. This arrangement worked very well for all of them, although they both said they were aware of some local criticism for taking this step. They discounted this criticism as 'jealousy at her getting the best of both worlds', but it remained as evidence of the way pressures to have children and for mothers to make the care of children their primary role are interlinked.

The Newsomes may speak for the joy these couples expressed:

> It took me a while to believe Paul was really there. It was unbelievable that we'd got a baby of our own at last. I'm still possessive with him and wrapped up with him. I don't think anyone else can look after him like me. Perhaps, later, I'll let go of him a bit. All the publicity about cot deaths frightened me; I was forever checking he was still breathing. I'd go off my head if anything happened to him. (Mrs Newsome)

> He's our special little miracle. We share him; all through I've taken a more active part than a lot of dads. (Mr Newsome)

> At the beginning it felt difficult to share him; first few weeks I was a bit selfish. Got a nice balance now. Cried quite a bit at first, when I was in hospital. I'd wanted him so much, but I was scared stiff. Had some post-natal depression at the start. (Mrs Newsome)

> We're just more protective than a normal couple would be. (Mr Newsome)

Three of the women said they had suffered from post-natal depression after the birth; Mrs Carver (who had DI), Mrs Newsome and Mrs Quick. Both Mrs Quick and Mrs Carver had been treated with drugs by their GP, and Mrs Quick was admitted to psychiatric hospital. Three out of 16 new mothers experiencing significant post-natal depression, two of whom required medication, is an unusually high figure (Welburn 1980, quotes an incidence of 10–18 per cent, and Stanway 1981, 10 per cent). Many approaches to understanding the dynamics of this problem, rather than the hormones, would readily explain the particular vulnerability of women who had emotionally invested so much in having a child. The significance of this finding would require testing in a much larger group. Whether or not the previous infertility is of etiological importance, there can be little doubt that it is important for the way the woman, her husband and those around her deal with the experience. The Carvers were adamant that DI had no bearing on her depression after the birth – denying that either of them had any doubts or regrets about the course taken. There was no evidence which might call this conviction into doubt.

The experience of the *Quicks* is of interest, in the particular pressures they experienced, wanting a child so much, and the birth bringing with it substantial *problems of parenthood*.

Mr Quick and his wife were in comfortable circumstances when referred to the Infertility Clinic. They were both in skilled jobs offering good earnings and security, and owned their own, very comfortable home. Pregnancy was for them the obvious next step. They impressed as a bright and articulate pair, she being the more forceful personality, who tended to lead in conversation, and he the calmer, more reflective, partner.

They attended the Infertility Clinic on only one occasion. Before she could go for the HSG, Mrs Quick was confirmed pregnant. They had been trying for a pregnancy for 22 months at the time of the first appointment. They both spoke strongly of the emotional pain that went with wanting to conceive without succeeding; the jealousy, and feelings of failure and bitterness. A month after the Clinic appointment she was admitted with a threatened miscarriage. This was averted and she gave birth normally.

Having experienced so little of the Infertility Clinic they had little comment to make beyond Mr Quick feeling rather annoyed that he had accompanied his wife to the Clinic, and to the GP, expecting to be treated as half of the 'problem', only to be completely ignored. They did gain a good enough impression of the concern of the staff and the time they took to listen to the patients, comparing it very favourably with the ante-natal clinic and his wife's treatment after giving birth.

> The after-care after having the baby was terrible – no time, not interested.

Mrs Quick spoke of how tired she became in hospital. From birth the baby, Alan, was very distressed and did not sleep. The rigid policy in the obstetric ward (not under the consultant who ran the Infertility Clinic) was for the babies to stay with the mother.

> They [the hospital staff] don't know anything about babies, that's the trouble. I was never given a break from him. No sleep for five days. I was in a terrible state when I got home. He cried and cried; they just left me. I lost my temper and shouted at him. Sister brought it up next day; never helped though, just made me feel guilty. He never slept, just cried and cried.

She was convinced there was something wrong with Alan, crying and being sick so much. Her mother, a health visitor, suggested it might be pyloric stenosis (an intestinal blockage). Only when Alan vomited so hard that he lost consciousness and had to be admitted to hospital were her fears taken seriously. The mother's suspicions were confirmed and he was operated on successfully. As he began to improve Mrs Quick deteriorated.

> Got him physically better, and I gave in. Washed out – getting no sleep . . . I hated Alan for a while. Felt guilty of having been to the Infertility Clinic, asked for help to get him, and yet still couldn't stand

sight of him . . . It was terrible, absolutely awful. I felt so bad; didn't realise I was depressed, thought I was going off my rocker.

Initially the GP tried antidepressants, then advised she went to stay with her parents to get help with Alan.

Didn't help; I ended up hating them as well as Alan. Got in a terrible state over going out anywhere. Got to the point of getting dizzy and blacking out, wandering off not knowing where I was going. I felt really bad; I'd hurt myself or the baby. Afraid if I touched him I'd kill him. Screamed at him.

Mrs Quick admits she used to believe that those with emotional problems should 'sort themselves out'; however, she remembered the futility of her mother-in-law saying 'buck yourself up'. Having been referred to a psychiatrist, a social worker visited her at home. Mrs Quick saw this as the turning point, when someone really listened to her desperation. She was admitted to the mother and baby psychiatric unit, with Alan, and the slow progress began. They were in-patients for six weeks, with their problems being treated as family ones (perhaps 'mothering' would be more accurate, as Mr Quick seems to have been little involved in the active treatment). Over a period of two months she gradually took up full responsibility for herself and Alan. She was unstinting in her praise for the psychiatric and social work service she received.

Although Mrs Quick saw her difficulty as being primarily one of hormonal imbalance, and was prescribed progesterone replacement during her next pregnancy, she also felt that the social context was important:

I blame the media for showing babies as so perfect . . . Society's changed – you're not living with your parents, you get no experience with babies either unless you've got younger brothers and sisters . . . The ante-natal clinic don't tell you what it's like; they never discuss problems like post-natal depression . . . We'd been looking forward to a baby so much – no one wanted a baby more than we did . . . They should talk a lot more about caring for a baby at home after discharge. The nurses don't help at all – only biology, that's no use . . . [Psychiatrist] said wanting it so badly could have made the post-natal depression worse.

With some misgiving, they tried for another child when Alan was almost 2, and conceived quickly. The second birth was not traumatic. They were much happier with the post-natal care of a different hospital, which accepted the mother's need for rest after the birth. Although she felt some resentment of her new baby, James, she now accepted this as a normal concomitant of the dependency of a small baby; accepted it and coped with it.

In retrospect they saw the experience as bringing them very much closer together as a couple, and causing them to value very highly having two healthy children.

This is another quite atypical case. However, the experience has more general application in warning of the importance that should be attached to the continuing care of someone who has sought help for infertility. The almost overwhelming feelings which can accompany childlessness may not entirely evaporate at conception. Something of the residue might, as in this case, appear to exacerbate the depression so commonly associated with the aftermath of childbirth.

By the time of the final interview, some of those who had conceived a child were thinking of trying for a second. This revived for all of them echoes of the first time.

Three of the couples had decided firmly that they were not prepared to consider investigations again.

> We'd like another baby, but haven't decided yet. We'd try for two or three years, but, if nothing happened, we'd give up. We've got one and anything else would be a bonus.　　　　　　　　　　(Mr Mitchell)

> I'd not go through all that again.　　　　　　　　　　(Mrs Mitchell)

For two couples there was a clear line in their minds, beyond which, at the time of our interview at least, they would not go.

> I'd probably take pills this time if necessary, but no more than that . . .
> We're not that desperate this time. Would like another, but wouldn't go along any of those paths again.　　　　　　　　　　(Mrs Butler)

The sense of being lucky was, not surprisingly, common to all of the couples.

> We wanted her so much, so happy with what we've got. I don't feel the necessity of another.　　　　　　　　　　(Mrs Coleman)

Not all of the couples felt the choice was entirely free, even this time.

> Still think there's as much pressure to have a second child as a first . . .
> I always said I'll be happy with one; I wanted a girl [*which they had*].
> Maybe I won't bother too much if I have problems; but now I'm not so sure.　　　　　　　　　　(Mrs Diamond)

The failure of the one-child family to gain popularity, despite an overall continued fall in completed family size (OPCS 1989), suggests that this pressure may be a reality for many parents in this position.

SUMMARY

Although not necessarily in as traumatic fashion as the initial experience of involuntary childlessness, it was clear from this study that the effects do not vanish with the birth of a child. The impact may be so severe and far reaching that support and sensitivity may be called for over an extended period. The available options to these couples for attaining parenthood have been discussed, and the particular demands they make. None of the options was without cost in some way.

None of the cases quoted in detail is claimed to be typical; rather, they demonstrate important considerations which sensitive services, both social and medical, should recognise for the involuntarily childless.

As was noted in relation to the impact of childlessness on marriage, it seems to be the case that the specific manner in which a couple seek to resolve their childlessness might not, of itself, carry additional threats to a relationship. The initial trials of infertility seem to have been the critical ones, in comparison with which these challenges are less threatening. This is, of course, not to diminish the importance of attending to their needs and concerns more sensitively than sometimes appears to be the case.

The primary aim of a medical service for infertility must be to enable the childless to have children. From the accounts of these couples the service studied was better than others discussed in the literature in being realistic with patients about the costs and benefits of further investigation and treatment. A much clearer understanding at the outset of the intentions of the couple, as well as the resources of the Clinic, would help an infertility service to respond more directly to the specific, and highly individual, needs of their patients. In this way the service could minimise the attrition of good-will caused by misunderstandings or plans which are not fully shared.

9 The present and the future

The pace of medical innovation has recently increased dramatically. Many dilemmas face those seeking help for their infertility; the studies reported in this book have suggested areas of particular concern.

SEEKING HELP FOR CHILDLESSNESS

There can be no doubt that all of those who might benefit from the investigation and treatment of infertility do not seek medical help. Equally, it must be the case that some couples never test their fertility, having decided to remain childfree.

The hidden childless

The choice of an urban, deprived working-class community for the study of rates of childlessness proved to be a significant one. Out of 1,166 ever-married women who took part in the survey, 16.9 per cent were found to be childless (could have conceived but had borne no live children) and just 2.1 per cent childfree (delaying conception or voluntarily childless). This suggested a rate of involuntary childlessness of 1:6, which was larger than other population estimates. It was anticipated that such an area, because of its class and age structure, might produce a rate in excess of a whole population rate. As with all other estimates of prevalence, this result must be taken as an indication which will only be properly tested by a thorough epidemiological study, which has yet to be undertaken in the UK.

Following the childless women responding to the initial GPS question-naire proved to be problematic for the reasons discussed in the text. Concentrating on those childless women still of reproductive age, the 19 per cent referred to above, showed some interesting characteristics. (Representing, as they did, a very small subsample of the practice population, demands that these be taken as indications for further research effort, rather than firm conclusions.) If these results were representative, then of the 19 per cent of women who 'could' have become pregnant, 45.2 per cent are postponing pregnancy, 45.2 per cent are involuntarily childless and 9.6 per cent are childfree. To express this in another way, for every thousand women under 45 in an urban working-class community, Table 9.1 indicates the groups which would be represented if these results were duplicated.

These figures must be regarded as estimates. It is to be hoped that they might stimulate further attempts to quantify this problem. The key point of interest to emerge in these figures is that, if this group medical practice is any guide, half of those women who want children but who are unable to conceive, do not ask to be referred on to hospital consultants.

It is well known that the true incidence of most medical complaints is well above that which comes to the attention of the hospital specialists, and even above that which comes to the attention of the general practitioner. The current climate of intense media and public attention to the advances in reproductive medicine, might encourage more to come forward of those who are not at the moment seeking investigation of their childlessness. This could result in a very substantial rise in the rate of referral. The recent advances, such as IVF, GIFT and ultrasound evaluation of ovulation, tend to be more expensive and time consuming than past methods. Having a birth rate which continues below replacement levels, has, perhaps, created the social conditions under which there is growing pressure to give priority to infertility than has hitherto been the case. The combination of these trends could make very considerable demands of scarce medical resources.

The voluntarily childless are a very small group according to these figures. In the light of other evidence, around 2 per cent is not likely to be an unreasonably low estimate, particularly in an urban, working-class area such as the one studied. Of all childless women, these figures suggest that

Table 9.1 Hypothesised distribution of childlessness[1]

Childfree		18
Delaying childbirth		86
Involuntarily childless:		86
of whom:		
seek specialist investigation	42	
only consult GP	12	
seek no help/advice	32	
Parous/have children		710
Total		1,000

1. Per thousand women co-habiting <45 years.

no more than one in ten will have elected not to have children, the others will have experienced fertility problems. Remaining childfree is still an unpopular choice.

A number of interesting factors were found in comparing the involuntarily childless with the childfree and the parous. The childless were older; also the apparent rate of childlessness amongst the over-45s was 1:5. With improved reproductive medicine and possibly wider acceptance of medical intervention, more women might be coming forward for help of this sort. A clear association was found between childlessness and social class. Almost twice the proportion of childlessness occurred amongst working-class as compared with middle-class women and working-class patients had an apparently high rate of non-referral for investigation. Delaying childbirth and being voluntarily childless, the childfree, was very clearly associated with social class – five times higher rates being found in the higher classes. Only one in five of the childless women was in employment compared with one in three of the mothers. This finding is at odds with the popular stereotype of the selfish, career-oriented childless woman some of the Clinic patients disliked but half-believed at the same time. There was little evidence of higher rates of separation and divorce amongst the childless women in the practice than the parous women: 13 per cent to 10.3 per cent. However, the limitations of the way in which these questions could be asked must make this interpretation tentative. Some evidence was also found that, in terms of self-reported serious illness and operations, the childless were more healthy than their parous sisters. This finding was not explained by the incidence of obstetric illnesses.

A not inconsiderable number of childless women do not currently seek medical help. This is important for the amount of unhappiness it represents, and also for the potential demand that might be created for specialist investigation in the future.

It is relevant to recall the characteristics of the childless couples who were seen in the Infertility Clinic at this point. They were not representative of the local community in certain respects. Ethnic minority people and those from religious minorities were very much under-represented. Better educated men were substantially over-represented; although this effect was not as marked amongst the women patients as the subjective impression of staff would have suggested. The lower social classes, as measured by occupation and council house tenancy, were very substantially under-represented. On this evidence, most of the patients were not predominantly articulate middle-class WASPs (White, Anglo-Saxon Protestants), as was the impression conveyed by a senior staff member, but there was a clear bias in that direction.

Both elements in this study have supported the view that infertility services are not evenly distributed across society; socially disadvantaged groups are more likely than the others to be found amongst the numbers of the hidden childless.

Seeking help

No clear evidence emerged concerning specific triggers which prompted people to be investigated for infertility. The picture given was that, having decided to try for children, failure quite soon felt very stressful. Many had in mind a 'reasonable' period of trying of several months or a year, after which they sought help from their GP. The key discriminating factors are perhaps those already discussed which appear to discourage some from seeking medical help beyond the GP. In that the couples in the study were rather older than might be expected, the delay in seeking specialist help was the more important. Some reluctance to seek the advice of the GP was evident. This first step seemed to be one taken with some difficulty by the couples interviewed. Almost half need the 'excuse' of another medical concern before raising the issue of childlessness. The general impression given was that the couples waited for the situation to become quite pressing: increased pressure from family and friends; growing personal distress; passing years. The step was not taken lightly or precipitately.

For many of these couples their infertility was borne with increasing concern until the point when their fear of being stigmatised publicly or ridiculed by family, friends or even doctor was overcome by the need to seek help. The personal significance of this step helps in understanding the apparently large numbers who fail to take it.

THE ROLE OF THE GENERAL PRACTITIONER

Some disparity emerged in the pictures drawn by the doctors themselves of how they expect to handle cases of infertility in their practice and the experience of the couples referred to the Infertility Clinic.

A high level of interest and concern was shown by the GPs questioned. There was very little evidence that the infertile were regarded, other than by a small minority, as a difficult group not commanding high priority for medical attention. Those who felt the subfertile commanded a priority that was 'rather low' or 'too low' clearly outnumbered those who felt that they are given too much priority.

The medical practice described suggested a willingness to become highly involved in the preliminary investigations and subsequent support of these patients. The situation described by the Clinic patients was less positive.

The principal concern with the Clinic couples was that the GP might have played a larger part in preparing them for the process of investigation. Whilst some basic investigation was done before referral on to the hospital, most doctors felt that it was a specialist matter. Consequently, the patients appeared not to have had an opportunity to anticipate the demands of investigation, and thus make an informed decision about proceeding.

There were substantial concerns about the operation of the Infertility Clinic from the perspective of the patients. One of the significant areas was the feeling that little trouble was taken by most of the doctors to explain what was happening; the investigations and treatments likely; the meaning of the results; the nature of the choices open to them. The GP, particularly if he or she has an established relationship with the patient, could play an important role in clarifying and explaining these matters. It appeared that the Clinic doctors were, on the whole, too busy, and the GPs thought it was the Clinic's responsibility (or at least made no contact with the patient), with the result that the couples were too often confused and unsure, and, in some cases, angry. This situation exacerbated the distress of the failure to conceive. If the GPs for these patients had undertaken the monitoring, supportive and counselling roles so many of the GPs surveyed envisaged, the patients would perhaps have had more positive views of the process they experienced. This would have involved the GP in making positive efforts to see the couple, who would not necessarily have come in the ordinary way. It must be accepted that busy GPs do not usually see themselves as able to invite more involvement than their patients themselves demand. It was not the case that these couples were taking the initiative to seek more support from their GP. This supportive and clarifying role might have been especially valuable at the point for some couples when they had not been helped to have a child, and they were facing significant choices for their futures.

It appeared that in many of the cases seen in the Infertility Clinic more might have been done about the 'basics' before referral. The lack of attention to sex in the investigations was one of these rather neglected basics. If GPs were able to help the couples in their practices to ensure that their sexual behaviour gave them the best possible chances of conception, not only might their progress, if referred on to a specialist, be enhanced, but some might not need to get that far, and others, unwilling to take that step, might still be helped.

The lack of involvement of many of the men has been a recurring theme. Unfortunately this began in the GPs' surgeries. As has been seen, very few GPs referred couples for investigation, although the majority of GPs responding to the survey claimed to take this course. Many never saw the man concerned at all. The GPs and the Infertility Clinic both seemed, by and large, to accept the prevailing social climate that all too readily allows the woman to shoulder the responsibility for infertility. Once a GP has felt it appropriate to refer only the woman for investigation, a pattern is established which may not easily change, whatever the expectations of the Clinic.

Most of these couples expressed satisfaction with the help they received from their GP, although perhaps not the usually high level of satisfaction most general studies in this area have produced. It seemed that GPs set themselves high standards for helping such patients which those in the study did not manage to attain. Other than when the exigencies of treatment required it (e.g. regular injections), there was little evidence that the GP felt that he or she was a member of a team treating the infertility. An awareness of the value in developing this concept of a team, which involved the doctor who would carry continuing responsibility for the care of the patient, led Froggatt (1982, 1983) to advocate the value of fertility co-operation cards in building a more structured role for the GP. Such a development would help to create this climate of joint care, and possibly improve the service received by the patient. The logistics of conveying very detailed and technical information might, however, make a card impractical, as the Clinic consultant argued. The strict regulations of the Human Fertilisation and Embryology Authority (HFEA 1991) forbid assisted reproduction services from routinely passing medical information to the patient's own GP, as is customary in all other secondary medical services. This could inhibit valuable co-operation.

It was encouraging that half of all the GPs in Sheffield were willing to complete an unheralded questionnaire on the subject – an unusually high response from GPs to any postal survey.

From the experience of these couples it would seem that their GP's support could be invaluable, particularly in the long intervals that punctuate investigation, and at times when crucial decisions have to be made about which options to pursue, or when to call a halt.

THE INFERTILITY CLINIC SERVICE

There was undoubtedly a high rate of criticism about the service provided by the Infertility Clinic at the time of this study. The dissatisfaction did seem excessive when compared with other surveys of hospital patients' opinions. Numerically, the complaints were twice as frequent as the complimentary comments made about the Clinic. However, this obscures a generally high opinion of the medical treatment itself, if not necessarily of the way in which it was delivered.

Several factors were likely to give this result: the high degree of emotional distress and intimate 'exposure' involved; asking opinions perhaps encourages expression of negative views more than positive ones; the under-funding and staffing difficulties this Clinic faced. In the light of the changes instituted since that time, it is likely that a much more favourable picture would now be obtained; however, it is also likely that many other infertility services would be subject to many of the same strictures applied in this case. It would be true to say that many of the concerns of these patients bore very little on the specific nature of their medical complaint, and would find echoes throughout the NHS hospital service. Very few of the patients involved in this study regretted having gone to the Infertility Clinic or would not have advised others to do the same. One source of increased complaint might well have been the disappointed 'customer'. As has been seen, those who remained childless were *not* more critical than those who were helped to have children.

The pregnancy rate amongst such a small sample of patients cannot be taken as valid for the whole service; 53 per cent would, however, seem a typical rate from the literature. There was a high degree of confidence amongst the couples that they would get the best possible treatment at this Clinic – scientifically and medically up to the minute with current developments. The one couple to take advantage of the private treatment in the University Clinic emphasised it was only in the expectation of a quicker, more efficient and personal service that they took the step, not in the hope of better medical care. No others had considered it, although there were a number who could easily afford it, and two who had undergone previous private medical treatment.

Gender differentials

The extent to which the woman was expected, by husband, Clinic and herself, to carry the heavier burden of investigation was striking. The many examples of the female orientation of the Clinic have already been cited. At one level this is not surprising for a service run by a department of obstetrics and gynaecology in a hospital for women. It did seem that a heavy price was thus exacted of the women, and a less efficient service run as a result.

The declared philosophy that infertility must be treated as a problem involving two people, whether or not the medical deficit was with just one of the partners, did not appear to be fully reflected in practice. A number of the men avoided contact from the beginning, at their own inclination, in response to the climate created by the appointment (letter, setting, specialty, etc.), or in response to their wife's views. In such cases, it seemed that the process was starting with a potential disadvantage. After the expenditure of considerable time and resources it could be that a couple would withdraw before a conclusion was reached. Investigation of the woman might be pursued in some depth where a major male problem was identified at an early stage. For a couple to pursue investigation and treatment in depth, the commitment of both husband and wife is important; in practice it seemed that the process often began with very little knowledge of the willingness of the husband to play the full part necessary. There was a clear difference between the policy of the Clinic set out by the consultant and the practice of the junior doctors, who, undertaking the initial investigations and examinations, were in a crucial position in setting the tone for the Clinic. Some of the concerns felt so deeply – e.g. lack of explanation, failing to understand the process – could have been ameliorated by having both husband and wife to hear results, ask questions, consider alternatives, etc.

One anomaly has been mentioned in relation to class expectations; it was of note in the study that the working-class couple with the clearest sexual problem (attitude and extreme infrequency) were neither given help by the Clinic staff nor referred on to a specialist service, although they attended the Clinic together and the husband made plain his willingness to be fully involved. The middle-class couple with severe marital problems which had a simple, recent sexual symptom (infrequent intercourse) found themselves referred on for specialist counselling, although the husband had not even attended the Infertility Clinic. A more consistent approach to the sexual aspect of the infertility presentation would be of value.

In the nature of reproductive medicine, the investigation and treatment of the woman is likely to be more protracted and demanding than that of the man. In itself this is an important reason for the organisation and approach of the Clinic to emphasise the essential role the husband is expected to play in the support of his wife. This is also a measure of his likely willingness to play a full part in treatment if a male problem is identified. No suggestion is being made that women should not have the right to decide the involvement their husband should have, if in fact the difficulty lies on her side. It is being argued that the Infertility Clinic, probably unwittingly, in various ways, colludes with attitudes that seem to accept that, whatever the emotional cost, the burden of infertility and its investigation should fall more heavily on the woman than the man, whatever the nature of the difficulty.

Organisation of the infertility clinic

The concerns about organisation and administration were set out in detail in Chapter 7. Some of the more unhelpful features of the original service have been rectified: the use of the ante-natal clinic; involvement of staff without a commitment to the problems of the subfertile; the gynaecological appointment card. Reactions of the few people in this study to experience the changes suggest that they have been well received.

In an under-funded service it is less easy to deal with issues such as inordinate waiting times, long gaps between appointments and changing doctors. It was clear that even these problems could be alleviated by clearer explanations of the process, and the constraints under which it operated. In the service which has been developed from the one studied here, the aim is to achieve assessment and diagnosis in a much shorter time. Waiting lists for operative procedures, notably laparoscopy, still cause significant delay.

The impact on the couples of initial and 'turning point' appointments was substantially different. The former set off with the barest introduction or explanation, with detailed history taking and physical examinations. Most couples felt very unprepared for this. Some felt that it was assumed that they were willing to undergo any investigation or treatment as long as it gave them a chance of conceiving a child. All of the couples would have welcomed a chance to have explained the implications of referral to the Clinic, and an opportunity to explain any limits they might see to their involvement; how far they might want to go. The notion of an initial 'contract' between the Clinic and the infertile couple would have started the process on a more positive footing.

The 'turning point' appointment was usually with the consultant, at which the findings were reviewed. It was usually the intention to explain either that nothing more could be done by the Clinic or that the next steps would involve a considerable investment of time and emotional energy, and possibly cash (e.g. IVF). This interview was without exception seen as helpful and caring, even where the news was bad, because of the trouble taken to explain the whole picture thoroughly, and give the time necessary to do this well. In a sense, it was very effective crisis intervention work. It was particularly welcomed that no attempt was made to 'string along' a couple with false hopes, rather to present the truth in a concerned but straightforward, adult fashion. If as much attention could have been given to the induction stage the couples might have felt substantially better about the whole process.

The in-patient care, usually for laparoscopy, was generally well regarded by the women in the study. The clear exception to this was the very unfortunate mixing of patients having abortions with those awaiting infertility-related procedures. Shortage of beds may make some of this unavoidable, but sensitivity to the feelings of the women involved would at least soften the experience. The more extreme insensitivity referred to in Chapter 7 cannot be excused. Such experiences lend weighty support to the challenge of Spallone (1989) that infertility services need to become person-led, not technique-led.

There was a substantial withdrawal rate from the Clinic; 27 per cent withdrawing from investigation before the Clinic indicated that there was no more help that could be offered. It is a difficult line to draw between premature withdrawal and the agreed termination considered in the 'turning point' interview mentioned above. In several of these cases a clear decision was made that the couple did not wish to go further. In two cases pregnancy followed anyway. There were few clear factors associated with the uni-lateral decision of patients to end investigation. The association with higher social class and close contact with families has been discussed. Although these findings were not the ones anticipated at the outset of this study, they perhaps serve to emphasise the vulnerable position in which these couples found themselves. Continuing investigation became increasingly painful for many of the couples, but the finality of withdrawing, involving accep-tance that they might never have children, could be even more painful. This might explain why the more articulate and better supported were more able to decide to withdraw. Investigation did become a treadmill that was very difficult to get off.

Six of the couples (20 per cent) were either in active treatment or on waiting lists for further help of some kind at the conclusion of the study – a period in excess of three-and-a-half years.

Overall many of the patients experienced the Infertility Clinic as a sympathetic and effective service. The substantial level of concerns did detract from this picture, with unfortunate consequences for the sense of involvement and commitment felt by the couples concerned.

After a period of unprecedented growth in infertility services, hard on the heels of the scientific explosion in knowledge of assisted reproduction techniques, there is increasing concern that expectations will not be matched by service realities. A political survey by Ms Harriet Harman of the Labour Party indicated the extent to which infertility services are unevenly distributed around the UK, and NAC claim that restrictions in spending on the National Health Service are leading to disproportionate cuts in these services (*Issue* 1991).

Alongside the media interest of the last few years and the scientific advances, Winston has been particularly outspoken in emphasising the gap between the promises and the delivery of babies to infertile couples, and the failures of general infertility services: he claimed to have found that only six patients in 150 referred on to him had received full and adequate baseline assessments (1990). He and feminist critics of the assisted repro-duction services point out that there are many dangers in heeding too soon the siren call of these 'glamorous' services. Preventive measures and treat-ment side effects are increasingly understood, but feature little in infertility services or media coverage (Klein 1989).

THE IMPACT OF CHILDLESSNESS

The experience of being involuntarily childless is profound and distressing.

Personal impact

With few exceptions, childlessness was described as an extremely upsetting situation, causing anguish, isolation and self-doubt. The perception that 'everyone', themselves included, expected them to have children left most of the couples with a 'spoiled identity'. In various ways they had to manage this stigma, often at the cost of isolating themselves from contact they would normally value, where it led to more questioning about their family intentions.

The conceptualisation of grief and bereavement is of value in understanding the variety of painful emotions many of them experienced, albeit grief without a visible object, and thus 'unfocused'. There was little evidence for a process of grieving in the stricter sense the literature sometimes envisages. All of the reactions described by Murray Parkes and others were evident at some stage.

Without exception, the people studied described surprise initially. The pronatalist assumptions of our society are so firm that the possibility that conception might not occur seems not to be anticipated, except in those cases where there has been a pre-existing medical condition known to impair fertility, e.g. oligomenorrhoea, testicular injury. Having had to guard against conception for so long, as many of the women saw it, by careful, planned contraception, impaired fertility had not been considered.

Denial might have been a factor that caused some of the couples in the study to delay seeking medical help for such a long period. Childlessness could not be something to affect them.

The isolation was very apparent. Very few of the couples were able to discuss their problems widely; some found it very hard even to talk to each other; many had not been able to confide in those to whom they would normally turn: parents, siblings, friends. This isolation contributed to the lack of preparation so many of them felt when embarking on investigation. The impact of peers and siblings having children increased the sense of isolation. They no longer shared central experiences, and the embarrassment and awkwardness of others made them turn away. Those who remained childless seemed to feel less able to cope with ordinary responsibilities and relationships than those who became parents.

Some of the anger directed towards the Clinic could well have had its origins in the anger aroused by the loss of fertility. The anger of those who had children might be considered an expression of the threat of loss which they experienced, although it turned out only to be temporary.

Strong feelings of guilt were expressed, exclusively by the women: guilt at the jealousy and envy aroused by the pregnancies of others; guilt at having taken the contraceptive pill for long periods, had an abortion or even dieted; guilt at not fulfilling the key internalised role demands for a wife to 'give' her husband a child. None of the men expressed feelings of guilt, not even those who were the only partner with a fertility deficit.

Depression was very strongly felt, again mainly by the women, who spoke poignantly of the hopelessness and helplessness of vainly striving for pregnancy. The increased demands, emotional and financial, of some of the new techniques of assisted reproduction might exacerbate this: it is suggested that three-quarters of those who are unsuccessful with IVF report depression (Mazure and Greenfeld 1989)

The move towards acceptance and resolution would be expected, but a number of different routes were involved. An even longer period of study would be required to see how those who were unsuccessful in having a child ultimately fared.

The extent to which the burden of the bad feelings was carried by the woman was very striking; particularly the way in which, with one exception, those women whose husbands were the ones with the fertility deficit took great pains to share the distress and to conceal the nature of the fertility problems. In several cases the woman was apparently happier to 'own the problem' rather than expect the husband to accept his responsibility. It was only men who conceptualised infertility as a threat to their image of themselves as men; none of the subfertile women spoke of feeling less feminine. There was no example of a husband shielding his wife by attempting to 'take the responsibility' for the infertility.

Whilst few of the patients confided widely over their difficulties, the men clearly talked less about the problems. The men said that they were less upset at their situation than their wives, and the measures used in the study confirmed this view in nearly all cases. Whilst the women wanting children spoke of their distress, guilt, bitterness and wishing to fulfil the role of wife, the men were more likely to express their feelings in terms of concern for their wife's distress, anger at the clinic system or distress at their own diagnosis of subfertility. None of the subfertile men spoke of a sense of failing to fulfil their role as husband. In no case did a couple declare that only the man was upset about the failure to conceive. The only people for whom antidepressant treatment was suggested were women. The distance many of the men were allowed to maintain between themselves and the Clinic investigations probably protected them in some measure. On average, the men became less anxious over time whatever happened; the women who remained childless did not.

There was a clear difference in the 'protective' effects of previous evidence of fertility. All of the men who had previously fathered a child saw that as reassurance to themselves. Their wives seemed to feel that it increased the pressure on them to fulfil their perceived role as wives, to 'live up' to the previous partner. The women who had had a previous pregnancy did not seem to feel this was any reassurance; all but one were terminated pregnancies which might have fuelled feelings of guilt. Whilst the Infertility Clinic, as part of the history taking, asked about previous terminations, it was unfortunate that this could simply increase the sense of guilt. Although current evidence suggests little connection between a properly conducted, early termination and subsequent infertility, Clinic staff did not appear to discuss this realistically with the women concerned.

The evidence available in this study gave no support to the idea that infertility is substantially caused by psychological or emotional conditions; there was no association between the level of anxiety, insofar as it was measured in this study, and the outcome of investigation and treatment. None of the unresolved situations remained entirely unexplained. There was, however, a great deal of evidence that the consequences of infertility were extremely distressing for most of the people in the study, especially the women. The very real pronatalist pressures described in this study seemed to bear most heavily on women. The evidence beginning to accrue suggests that the complexity of assisted reproduction techniques and, in some cases, their very nature – e.g. selective reduction of embryos after IVF – will increase the emotional demands on infertile people in treatment, particularly the women.

Effects on the marriage

'Crisis' is an appropriate term with which to describe the effects of child-lessness. Few of the couples felt that the experience had no impact on their relationship, although a range of reactions was described.

The majority of couples felt that, in some respects, the investigations themselves adversely affected the relationship. Chief amongst these factors was the difficulty experienced in the sexual relationship. Although the Clinic staff appeared to raise the matter of sex as little as possible, most of the couples felt that their sexual relationship suffered temporarily. The common complaint was the feeling that it became exclusively focused on conception, was artificial and lacked spontaneity. Most of the couples, with the exception of those who separated, saw this effect as temporary and improving when they either conceived or accepted that they would not have children. Some couples reported an improvement in their sex lives on stopping regular BBT charts. The relationship was described as taking a long time to return to normal.

The marriages of those who remained childless appeared on average to involve more joint relationships, and possibly to be more egalitarian, than those with children. The explanation for this must include the effects of children on the other relationships, pushing them towards more segregated roles. There was some evidence that amongst those who remained childless the men appeared to feel less positive about the marriage than the women. However, in most cases – those who had children and those who did not – they were likely to describe their marriage as being closer, with the clear exception of those whose marriages foundered. Both of the marriages that did not last had clear tensions which only in part involved infertility. In one case the childlessness appeared to prompt the wife into a fairly fundamental reassessment of her expectations of marriage, and indeed her life. In the other, this particular tension raised questions about the husband's priorities and willingness to compromise his wishes with those of his wife. In both situations the childlessness was a crisis that called into question some taken-for-granted matters concerning the marriage and relationship. In both cases the man showed himself unwilling to change or make compromises which would recognise the turmoil being experienced by the woman. For both women, conception had been an unquestioned and essential component of the way they saw themselves and the marriage. Both men took the minimum part in the investigation demanded of them. Neither had expected to share the experience with their wives, whatever the diagnosis.

Just as it was several times pointed out that children will not cement an ailing marriage, others emphasised that weathering the storms of infertility and its investigation was a severe test of a relationship; a true crisis in Caplan's terms. The marriages that survived were mostly felt to have been strengthened as a result by the sense of common purpose forged in adversity.

Effects of children

Over half of the couples in the study were successful in having a child, most of them after treatment. None of the births was multiple – one of the much publicised consequences of some infertility treatment. All of the children born were healthy. One woman suffered an ectopic pregnancy, but there were no other major birth problems.

The cases of post-natal depression were discussed in some detail in the text. Whilst 3 in 16 appears to represent an unusually high incidence, the small size of the sample must be remembered. Each of the women, not surprisingly given the purpose of the interview, made the link with the preceding investigations. This is a matter that could be considered further with advantage, particularly as one conceived through DI. There is no indication in the literature concerning DI that such births, insofar as it has been possible to study them, are especially likely to carry a risk of post-natal depression.

Although the evidence gathered was impressionistic, there was little that the children themselves were unduly cosseted. All of the parents spoke very warmly of their children, but without evidence of serious over-protectiveness. Many of the same anxieties and feelings of pressure were expressed in relation to the decision about having another child. To these feelings were now added the concerns as to whether they were able or willing to tread the same path again to have another child.

Childlessness had a very major effect on nearly all of the couples in this study. It constituted a crisis which tested their coping mechanisms to the full. For nearly all of the couples, infertility was seen as a painful but survivable experience, as a result of which they knew each other and their relationship better.

Meeting the emotional needs of infertile couples

In practice, the couples in this study had very little contact with counsellors or social workers. Those who considered adoption were the main exception. One woman also related very positive contacts with a psychiatric social worker over her post-natal depression. The only other formal counselling encountered was that offered as part of the DI service; this was undertaken by a marriage guidance counsellor or a doctor.

The social work department had very little contact with the Infertility Clinic, although it was apparent that they were fully aware of the needs of the couples concerned and the way the service failed to meet some of those needs. The pressure of competing demands limited their involvement. The potential contribution of social workers and other helping professionals to an infertility service might be summarised in several areas. In some of the areas other professional staff might, of course, be in a position to offer similar services.

Counselling

The term is used here in a generic sense, in which it is intended to convey that interpersonal helping process for individuals and families which focuses on feelings and relationships. The same sense might be conveyed in the term 'casework' or 'psychotherapy', particularly as this latter term was used in some of the literature discussed in Chapter 2. Counsellors are increasingly being appointed in infertility clinics, particularly in association with such assisted reproduction services as DI, IVF and GIFT. The

Warnock Commission and the Interim Licensing Authority played a significant role in getting counselling to be recognised as an essential part of the multi-disciplinary service couples require. This has now been made a requirement of infertility services which offer DI and IVF (although, curiously, not GIFT) under provisions of the Human Fertilisation and Embryology Act 1990. A new association has been informed to promote such services and enhance their quality: the British Infertility Counselling Association (BICA). Neither the legislation itself nor the associated Code of Practice (HFEA 1991) makes any requirements as to the qualifications of those providing the counselling. The pace of development in this area has been rapid since the time of the fieldwork reported here.

Bereavement counselling has become a recognised, valuable service, often offered by social workers in hospital settings. In the light of the analogy with loss discussed here, this approach could be of considerable value in this context. Although only one-third of the couples raised the potential value of a counselling service, a number chose to say how much they valued the opportunity for reflection in the research interview. It was a non-threatening situation, in which the couple were encouraged to talk about their feelings, in an open-ended interview which guaranteed confidentiality, with someone offering time and empathic, non-judgemental 'active listening'. This situation was quite a close analogy to a counselling service, although not designed for that purpose or perceived as such by most of the interviewees. A couple, such as the Truswells discussed in detail in Chapter 8, would probably reject out of hand the opportunity of counselling as such, but an explanatory or introductory interview offered by a social worker or counsellor could have offered this same experience, which they clearly valued. The HFEA Code of Practice refers to this as implications counselling.

Gender issues also arise in this context. It is often noted, as discussed in Chapters 6 and 7, that men are less easy to engage in counselling than women. These findings have major implications for how well men are likely to make use of counselling services in the Infertility Clinic. It is essential that such services take account of these general trends, alongside the particular concerns raised in this study.

A counsellor who was clearly seen as part of the Clinic team would be able to offer this service as a 'normal' aspect of the process, rather than as a potentially, stigmatised service for the non-copers. It is to be hoped that the counselling offered under the Human Fertilisation and Embryology Act's Code of Practice will not be confined as narrowly to the procedures currently specified.

Consultancy

An awareness of the feelings and experiences of couples undergoing infertility investigation was evident in the comments of the medical social workers quoted in Chapter 7. In their knowledge of groupwork methods and the contribution of self-help groups, social workers are well placed to facilitate the development of such opportunities for those couples who would find it helpful. Such groups might have information and explanation as central functions, and would inevitably offer valuable peer support if well handled by a skilled 'leader' or facilitator. Nursing staff might be well placed to 'run' such groups. Social workers could helpfully advise on their organisation to avoid the groups being simply passive, 'led' groups stifling self-help and open sharing of painful feelings. This Infertility Clinic has begun to operate such a service with nursing staff.

Many of the concerns voiced about the operation of this infertility service related to patients feeling that their emotions were neither considered nor understood. A team counsellor or social worker would be in a position to act as spokesperson and advocate to other staff; identifying factors in the service which were particularly inhibiting or undermining.

Donor insemination

Skilled counselling is now recognised by statute as an essential component of a DI service. No attempt was made to assess the counselling available in the two services involved in this study. Certain comments might be made about the focus of such a service. Making an assessment of the joint commitment to the treatment is a major factor, and that the relationship appears strong enough to withstand any reactions of jealousy or envy that might occur. The counsellor has to ensure that the couple fully understand the nature of DI and its implications. What seem often to be ill-considered are the issues of secrecy and confidentiality discussed in Chapter 8. All of the couples in the study appeared to have opted for a scenario that as few people as possible would be told, and that the child would probably not be told. Adoption workers have gained acceptance for the value to the child's sense of identity as well as the relationship between 'parent' and child, of having the child's origins open and discussed from earliest times. This view received official endorsement in the Department of Health consultation document (1990). The Human Fertilisation and Embryology Act requires such openness in the future, giving adults conceived through DI the right to information about their genetic parentage, after counselling. The Act specifically rules out retrospection, in contrast to adoption legislation, so that children conceived at the time of this study would not be affected.

There was, however, no evidence from this study that DI itself threatens marriages. For most of the couples it seemed that the testing times had been the investigation, coming to terms with the diagnosis and making the decision to attempt DI. This might be when help should be available to assist couples in looking at the emotional implications of their situation. By the time the couple have reached the DI clinic much of the emotional work may have been done, and possibly decisions taken about matters like 'telling', which will not then be easily changed.

Adoption and fostering

There is a clear need for medical and nursing staff to be well informed on the nature of these services, the availability of children, the process of assessment and the agencies involved. Whilst there was little evidence of erroneous information being received by patients in this study, it seemed that the implications of strict age limits were not informing as fully as necessary the practice of the Clinic and advice given to the couples. Couples were, however, aware of the situation.

The distinction between fostering and adoption seemed clear for all of those interviewed, despite the confusion evident in some of the medical literature. Clarification might be essential for some infertility services.

The ambivalence of these services towards the childless couple has been pointed out. It was argued that the unhappy experiences of the Greens were in part associated with this. An adoption service must see itself as choosing suitable homes from the many offered for the few children available; a fostering service must be concerned to recruit families for the many children in need of substitute care. The tensions of demand and supply can lead to the neglect of the emotional difficulties of the childless couple, which have been extensively discussed in this study. This must be to the detriment of both the needs of children and the childless couples.

There is a sound case to be made for a social work input to infertility services to ensure that these insights and skills are available both to staff and the couples themselves, who are engaged on such an emotionally demanding and uncertain course.

Childlessness is a burden borne by a considerable number of couples; few of whom obtain the support they need because of their isolation in our pronatalist society. The rapid expansion of assisted reproduction techniques must be seen as a two-edged sword: it offers hope, but demands considerable emotional stamina and resilience from the infertile couple and, especially, the woman involved. Medical and social services need a clear understanding of the personal and social pressures experienced by involuntarily childless people. This will enable these services to be more sensitive and responsive to their feelings and more able to help them cope effectively. The challenge for all of these services is to offer childless people informed and realistic choice.

Appendix I: Glossary of medical terms

Note: This is intended primarily as a guide to terms used in the text, and not as a comprehensive list of all conditions, tests and treatments relevant to the infertile. Principal references used in compiling this glossary are Stangel (1979), Menning (1977) and Winston (1986 and 1990) with the additional advice of Professor I.D.Cooke.

Abortion	Premature loss of developing foetus; in lay use confined to artificially induced loss; in medical use both spontaneous (miscarriage) and induced (TOP); (see also early abortion).
Adenomyosis	Abnormal growth of endometrium in the wall of the uterus, instead of in the lining, its normal site, like endometriosis *q.v.*
Adhesion	Abnormal attachment of adjacent membranes by bands or masses of fibrous connective tissue which grow in a damaged area; frequently caused, and correctable, by surgery; may block or immobilise tubes, uterus or ovaries.
AID	See *Donor insemination*.
AIDS	Acquired immuno-deficiency syndrome.
AIH	By mechanical means, placing husband's semen in the vagina (sometimes uterus) to achieve conception; used in cases of mucus hostility, poor coitus, or poor sperm quality.
Amenorrhoea	Absence of menstruation.
Anastomosis	Microsurgical removal of blocked or diseased section of fallopian tube or vas deferens and rejoining of healthy ends.
Andrology	(*Medical*) Science of diseases in male reproductive system.

Anovulation	Total failure of ovulation; *note* not the same as amenorrhoea, apparently normal menses may continue.
Asynchronous cycle	Menstrual cycle in which the hormone secretion does not match the required pattern, typically the LH surge does not coincide with follicle ripening in order for egg to be released.
Azoospermia	Absence of sperm in the semen; sterility.
BBT	Basal body temperature, charted by woman at same time each day (usually on waking) when suspected of failing to ovulate correctly; provides secondary evidence of the release of essential hormones; normal chart is biphasic, temperature usually drops immediately before ovulation, rises immediately afterwards, and stays up until the period starts; a routine but inexact test.
Bicornuate uterus	Congenital deformity of the womb in which the 'corners', where the fallopian tubes enter, are drawn out like horns, and the uterus is divided by a wall (septum) down the middle to some extent (completely in rare cases); the relevance of this condition to infertility is controversial, but thought to be particularly significant where there is subseptate or incomplete division.
Biopsy	Surgical removal, then microscopic examination, of a piece of living tissue; in infertility, particularly for the assessment of sperm production (testicular), ovulation (ovarian) and womb function (endometrial).
Bromocriptine	Trade name Parlodel; inhibits prolactin secretion by pituitary, which in excess (hyperprolactinaemia) inhibits ovulation.
Capacitation	Alteration of the spermatozoa during its passage through the female reproductive tract during which full maturity is reached, enabling penetration and fertilisation of the ovum.
Cervix	Neck or opening of uterus into vagina.
Chlamydia	Pathogens which may cause infection of the fallopian tubes.
Clomid	See *Clomiphene*.
Clomiphene	Trade name, Clomid. Most commonly used drug

	to stimulate ovulation; pills given for 5 days near start of cycle.
Coitus	Act of sexual intercourse.
Corpus luteum	Special gland which forms in the ovary at the site of ovulation, the follicle, and produces progesterone; characteristic of second half of cycle and essential for preparation of the endometrium for implantation of the embryo.
Curettage	See *D & C.*
D & C	Dilatation and curettage, dilating cervix to admit instrument to the uterus to scrape its lining and, often, take endometrial biopsy.
DI	See *Donor insemination.*
Danazol	Trade name Danol; treatment for endometriosis, synthetic androgen, causes cessation of ovarian activity through pituitary (conception therefore impossible during Danazol therapy).
Defective luteal phase	Failure of progesterone level to rise after ovulation thus preparing the uterus for implantation.
Dilatation	See *D & C.*
Dizygotic	Of twins, simultaneous development of two fertilised ova.
Donor insemination	Using mechanical means to place donor semen in the vagina (sometimes uterus) to achieve conception; used in cases of inadequate sperm or sterility of the partner; *N.B.* previously known as AID.
Dysmenorrhoea	Painful menstruation.
Dyspareunia	Pain experienced during sexual intercourse.
Early abortion	Loss of the embryo shortly after fertilisation and before implantation; may not be detected easily.
Ectopic pregnancy	Embryo implants in tube instead of uterus, and subsequently aborts (or is aborted); may leave substantial scarring or blockage of tube, which is thus impaired.
Ejaculation	Male orgasm during which semen is ejected.
Embryo transfer	Return of fertilised egg to uterus during IVF.
Endocrinology	(*Medical*) Scientific study of hormone-producing system.
Endometriosis	Development of tissue-like endometrium outside

the uterus which may cause infertility (controversial); treated with progestogens or Danazol.

Endometrium — Lining of the uterus.

Epididymis — Long coiled tube carrying sperm from testis to vas deferens and thus exit, in which vital maturation of the sperm takes place.

Fallopian tube — (*Salpinx*) Pair of fine tubes running from top of uterus to terminate near the ovary, where sperm fertilise ovum and first 3–4 days of development of the embryo occurs during transport to uterus and implantation in the endometrium.

Ferning test — A procedure in which a sample of mucus is dried on a slide and examined under the microscope; the degree of ferning increases with the oestrogen content, and is inhibited by progesterone.

Fertilisation — Penetration of ovum by a sperm.

Fibroid — Benign tumour of fibrous tissue in the uterine wall; may cause menstrual and infertility problems; removal by myomectomy, which itself may inhibit fertility through tissue scarring and resultant adhesions.

Follicle — Cavity or blister in the ovary within which the egg develops; lined with the granulosa cells which produce first oestrogen and then progesterone.

FSH — Follicle stimulating hormone; secreted by pituitary; controls (with LH) ovulation in women and sperm production in men; extracted from the urine of post-menopausal women; a highly effective, expensive recent alternative to HMG with similar function.

Gamete — Male (sperm) or female (ovum) reproductive cells.

GIFT — Gamete intra-fallopian treatment; technique in which eggs and sperm are mixed and returned immediately to the fallopian tube; also known as T-SET (tube–sperm–egg transfer).

Gonads — Sex glands that produce the gametes; testis in the male, ovary in the female.

Gonadotrophins — Pituitary hormones, LH and FSH *q.v.*

GnRH — Gonadotrophin-releasing hormones; naturally produced by hypothalamus to cause pituitary

	gland to release LH and FSH; in synthesis can be given by pulse pump.
Gynaecology	(*Medical*) Science of diseases in women.
HCG	Human chorionic gonadotrophin; hormone secreted by the placenta in pregnancy to prolong life of the corpus luteum. Similar to hormone LH, may be given by injection around 14th day of cycle to encourage follicle to release egg.
HMG	Human menopausal gonadotrophin, trade name Pergonal; the 'fertility drug'. Purified natural combination of LH and FSH, powerful stimulator of egg production; by injection in carefully controlled dosage for several days in first half of cycle. Carries serious risk of multiple ovulation.
HSG	Hysterosalpingogram; X-ray examination of fallopian tubes whilst dye is being inserted, to assess their patency, i.e. capacity to carry dye along the length until spilling freely into the abdominal cavity at the free (fimbrial) end near the ovary.
Hydrosalpinx	Fluid trapped in the fallopian tube, usually implying occlusion of the tube.
Hymen	Membrane covering the opening of the vagina normally broken by penis at first full intercourse.
Hyperprolactinaemia	Excess levels of prolactin in the bloodstream which inhibit ovulation.
Hypogonadism	Atrophy or reduction of the gonads.
Hypospadias	Opening of the urethra is below the shaft of the penis, not at the tip.
Hypothalamus	The part of the brain that secretes releasing hormones which stimulate production of LH and FSH by the pituitary.
Hysteroscopy	Visual examination of the uterus using a slim, illuminated 'telescope', the hysterocope; inserted via the vagina, usually under anaesthetic.
IUD	Intra-uterine contraceptive device, the coil or loop, may be a cause of PID and thus infertility.
IUI	Intra-uterine insemination: artificial insemination of ovum within the uterus.
IVF	*In vitro* fertilisation; extra-corporeal fertilisation (i.e. out-of-body or 'in glass'). Surgical extraction of ripe egg(s) (ovum) from the ovary, fertilisation

	with semen in laboratory dish containing a culture medium and replacement of developing embryo at *c.* 2 days old in the uterus.
Immunological factors	Presence of sperm antibodies in the woman or man that tend to destroy the sperm's action by immobilising them or making them clump together.
Implantation	Attachment of the fertilised ovum to the endometrium.
Inadequate sperm	Lay description of sperm which are below viable limits of motility, morphology, number or progression.
Insufflation	(*Rubin test*) blowing gas through the fallopian tubes to assess patency; losing favour for pain caused and results of limited value.
Laparoscopy	Examination of abdominal cavity, thus principal female sex organs, by a slim, illuminated medical 'telescope', the laparoscope; inserted through incision in the abdomen, normally done under general anaesthetic.
Laparotomy	Abdominal surgery.
Ligation	Tying off in surgery.
Luteal phase	Days 12–18 of normal menstrual cycle.
Luteinizing hormone	(LH) Produced by pituitary gland; controls (with FSH) ovulation in women and sperm production in men.
Maturation defect	Failure of sperm to develop fully prior to ejaculation.
Menarche	Onset of menstruation in girls.
Menopause	Cessation of menstruation due to ageing or failure of the ovaries, normally occurs between 40 and 50 years; also called 'change of life'.
Mensis	(*pl. menses*) Menstrual period.
Menstruation	Cyclic bleeding that normally occurs every 26–29 days in mature non-pregnant female until menopause; bleeding caused by the loss of the endometrium.
Microinsemination	Insertion of sperm directly into the ovum using microsurgical techniques.
Microsurgery	Surgery using microscope, particularly valuable in tubal surgery.
Mittelschmerz	(*lit. 'middle pain'*) Experienced by some women around the time of ovulation, i.e. in mid-cycle.

Monozygotic	Of twins, development of two embryos from single fertilised ovum, therefore genetically identical.
Morphology	Structure of individual sperm; measured as proportion of normal to abnormal forms.
Motility	Ability of the sperm to move in progressive, linear fashion; recent innovations in assessment include the swim-up and velocity tests which quantify this ability.
Mucus	Jelly-like body fluid produced by the cervix, in greater quantities and more watery at the time of ovulation than at other times of the cycle.
Myomectomy	Operation for removal of fibroids *q.v.*
Nulliparous	Not having borne a child previously.
Obstetrics	(*Medical*) Scientific study of childbirth.
Oedema	Fluid retention in tissues.
Oestrogen	Hormone produced by specialised cells (granulosa) in the follicle, encourages uterus to grow and the lining (endometrium) to thicken.
Oligomenorrhoea	Irregular, few or scanty periods.
Oligospermia	Fewer than normal sperm; sometimes also with inadequate progression and increased number of abnormal forms; range of 'normal' is controversial, in this Clinic less than 20 million sperm per ml semen considered abnormal.
Orgasm	Moment of peak sexual excitement at which semen is ejaculated in man, and climax is experienced by female with strong contractions of the uterus.
Ovary	Female sexual gland produces oestrogen and progesterone, and eggs (ova).
Oviduct	Fallopian tube.
Ovulation	Release of mature ovum from follicle on surface of ovary.
Ovum	(*pl. ova*) female gamete, egg.
Parous	Having borne a child.
Pelvic inflammatory disease	(*PID*) Salpingitis, later chronic disease or consequent damage, frequent cause of tubal disease and adhesions.
Pergonal	See *HMG*.
Pituitary gland	The controlling gland in the brain, produces key hormones for sexual development, LH and FSH,

which act on the ovaries in women to stimulate ovulation, and the testes in men to produce sperm.

Plasma progesterone measurement	Test of level of progesterone in blood, raised levels usually indicate ovulation has occurred.
PCO	Polycystic ovarian disease; ovaries develop numerous small cysts inside preventing normal function.
Polyp	Nodule or small, benign growth often found on mucous membranes such as cervix or uterus.
PCT	Post-coital test; examination of cervical mucus sample 6–24 hours after intercourse to assess survival and progressive movement of sperm (also called Hühner or PK Test).
Pre-eclamptic toxaemia	Pregancy disease of weight gain, oedema and hypertension.
Progesterone	Hormone produced by cells in the developing corpus luteum which stimulates the glands of the endometrium in preparation for implantation of fertilised egg.
Puberty	Time of life when male and female reproductive organs become fully functional.
Puerperium	(Period of) childbirth.
Pump therapy	See *GnRH*.
Retrograde ejaculation	Muscular fault causing sperm to be ejaculated into bladder at orgasm rather than outside via urethra.
Retroverted uterus	Uterus is tilted backwards, occurs in *c.* 25 per cent women, recent evidence suggests this is not in itself a cause of infertility as previously believed.
Salpingitis	Infection of salpinx (fallopian tube).
Salpingolysis	Operation to free tubes of adhesions.
Salpingostomy	Operation to open blocked tube.
Salpinx	Fallopian tube.
Semen	Sperm mixed with seminal fluids produced in the seminal vesicles and prostate gland to comprise the ejaculate.
Semen analysis	Microscopic examination of a semen sample to determine the quantity of the semen and quality of the sperm, i.e. motility (ability to move forward), morphology (proportion of normal to abnormal forms), and number (count of sperm present per ml semen).

Seminal vesicle	Reservoir connected to vas deferens which produces jelly-like fluid to carry sperm.
Seminiferous tubules	Long tubes in the testis in which the sperm are formed.
Sperm antibodies	Antibodies develop to protect the body against invasion by foreign matter such as bacteria; may develop in the cervix of some women against partner's sperm, or even in some men killing their own sperm.
Sperm test	See *Semen analysis.*
Spermatogenesis	Production of sperm in the seminiferous tubules.
Spermatozoa	Synonym for sperm.
Split ejaculate	Technique of collecting first part of ejaculate separately which contains most of the sperm.
Stein–Leventhal syndrome	Also known as PCO *q.v.*
T-SET	Same as GIFT *q.v.*
Tamoxifen	Similar to clomiphene.
Temperature chart	See *BBT.*
Test tube treatment	See *IVF.*
Testis	(*pl. testes*) Male sexual gland (testicle) produces testosterone and male reproductive cell, sperm.
Testosterone	Principal male sex hormone produced in the testes.
TOP	Termination of pregnancy, i.e. induced abortion.
Toxaemia	(*Colloq*) Infection of the blood. See *Pre-eclamptic toxaemia.*
Tubal disease	Fallopian tubes with partial or complete blockage, damage to the lining or muscle wall, or adhesions; in each case these conditions limit ability of tube to carry ova and sperm effectively to enable fertilisation and implantation in uterus; microsurgery is only treatment, still of limited efficacy.
Tubal spasm	Muscular spasm of the fallopian tubes, which probably inhibits transport of sperm and ovum and fertilisation.
Tubal reanastomosis	Surgical rejoining of fallopian tubes ligated (cut and tied) for sterilisation.
Turner's syndrome	Genetic abnormality in which female has XO chromosomes instead of normal XX; most such women are sterile.

Ultrasound	Machine based on sonar to give visual image of bodily organs by the reflection of sound waves; widely used in monitoring of ovulation and assessment of reproductive organs.
Urethra	Tube connecting bladder to outside, also final pathway for sperm and semen.
Urology	(*Medical*) Scientific study of male reproductive tract and male or female urinary tracts.
Uterus	Synonym for womb.
Vagina	Passage connecting female external sex organs with cervix and uterus; accommodates penis in coitus.
Vaginismus	Muscular spasm of the vagina, making penetration by the penis painful or even impossible.
Varicocele	Enlargement of veins around the testis; may cause impaired sperm production because of temperature increase.
Vas deferens	Tube carrying sperm from epididymis to urethra, muscular walls important in propelling semen at ejaculation.
Vasectomy	Minor surgery to ligate (cut and tie) vas deferens; male sterilisation procedure.
Vasogram	X-ray of male reproductive tract during the infiltration of radio opaque dye, in order to demonstrate constriction or obstruction of the tubes.
Venereal disease	Any infection transmitted by sexual intercourse; most common forms are syphilis and gonorrhoea; untreated, an important and increasing cause of infertility.
Zona penetration test	Test of the ability of the sperm to penetrate the zona pellucida, the protective layer around the ovum; uses hamster eggs or separated human zonas from a fertilised ovum.

Appendix II: Normal reproduction

There is now a substantial number of lay guides to the processes of reproduction; several of them written specifically for the childless. Because of the recent pace of scientific development, the fine detail becomes out of date quite quickly. Amongst the more useful are Stangel (1979), Stanway (1984), and Winston (1986 and 1990).

A simplified and abbreviated account of the normal reproductive process is given here, in order to elucidate the text. More detail may be obtained from the references given. It should be remembered that what will be described is essentially a statistical norm; that is the way things occur in most people. There is significant variation between individuals in matters such as length of menstrual cycle and quantity of sperm produced. This variation may not be pathological nor impede fertility.

Essentially, conception involves the meeting of sperm and egg in suitable conditions. In both male and female, the organs of reproduction are paired up to the single urethra in men and single uterus in women.

SPERM PRODUCTION

Spermatozoa or sperm are first produced at puberty, prompted by hormones secreted by the pituitary gland, LH and FSH. Sperm production is also called spermatogenesis. They form in the testis or testicle, the male sex organ (gonad), which hangs in the scrotum. This siting is required because the sperm require a temperature some four degrees below body heat to develop normally. The sperm's development continues in a series of ducts; the rete testis, efferent ducts and epididymis. Only when they reach the vas deferens are they fully formed. The vas deferens is the muscular tube which transports sperm to the urethra, in the process being mixed with seminal fluid secreted from the seminal vesicles and prostate gland. This fluid provides a transport medium for the sperm, but is also essential for the health of the sperm during this period. At orgasm, the vas deferens contracts strongly to force the semen on into the urethra whence it is ejaculated by muscular action of the penis. The process of sperm production takes 2–3 weeks. Even at this stage the sperm are not fully functional; chemical changes are required, called capacitation, which occur on contact with the woman's body fluids.

A normal male produces some 100 million spermatozoa each day.

EGG PRODUCTION

At birth, the woman's ovaries contained the full complement of eggs (ova), some two million. At puberty the ovary is stimulated into action by the hormones LH and FSH produced in the pituitary, which will continue to govern the process of egg production throughout the woman's active reproductive life. A pocket or follicle develops around an egg to nurture it; stimulated by FSH it produces oestrogen. Once a month, FSH secretions (in part) cause one of the follicles to develop strongly, leaving others to wither away. The oestrogen it produces causes the uterus to grow in size and its lining, the endometrium, to thicken and develop glands necessary to nourish sperm and ovum which might be received. Under the control of gonadotrophin-releasing hormones from the hypothalamus, the pituitary produces a surge of LH which triggers the rupture of the follicle, ovulation. The follicle changes chemical action, now producing oestrogen and progesterone; the ruptured follicle takes on a yellow colour, becoming known as the corpus luteum. Only if conception occurs will this continue beyond 14 days or so. The ovulated egg is collected by the fringed (fimbrial) end of the fallopian tube.

MENSTRUATION

Menstruation is the sign of failure to conceive, and occurs approximately monthly. It is not necessarily an indication of ovulation. Menstruation may occur without ovulation, and vice versa. Menstrual bleeding is the shedding of the fragmenting lining of the womb, the endometrium. Having been prepared for the reception of the fertilised egg, as described above, the enlarged endometrium is not required if conception does not occur and is therefore shed some 14 days after ovulation. This process takes some five days and is triggered by the fall in secretion of progesterone. The cycle is measured from the first day of menstrual bleeding.

FERTILISATION

At intercourse, the man ejaculates between 100 and 800 million sperm in 1 to 8 millilitres of semen into the vagina of the woman. These quantities naturally vary between men and also at different times in the same man, quite independent of artificial interference. The fertility of the semen principally depends on the morphology, motility and progression as well as the number of sperm present; these are the factors measured in semen analysis.

Many of these sperm trickle outside the vagina after withdrawal. Most remain just inside the vagina, dying rapidly from the acidic environment. A small proportion, at most a few million, move on through the cervical mucus at the neck of the uterus. This mucus changes character in response to the menstrual cycle, becoming copious and watery just before the time of ovulation, thick and scanty at other times. Only within a period of four or five days before ovulation is the mucus hospitable to sperm. At this time they may swim through the mucus into the uterus, being released regularly over a period of time. Once the mucus begins to thicken and decrease they become immobilised and die. From the uterus sperm enter the tubes. This appears to be achieved by a combination of the sperm's own motility, a pumping action of the uterus (possibly enhanced by the woman's orgasm), and negative pressure in the tubes. Sperm can reach the fallopian tube as soon as 15 minutes from intercourse. Sperm can survive in the tube for several days. Some of the sperm will progress along the tube to the fimbrial end near which fertilisation may occur with a ripe ovum. Only one sperm can successfully fertilise the ovum.

EMBRYO DEVELOPMENT AND IMPLANTATION

The fertilised egg develops in the tube for the first 92 hours, and divides several times as it is carried back to the uterus. When it enters the uterus the embryo consists of some 64 cells. This embryo may float around the uterus for 2 or 3 days before attaching to the lining of the womb, the endometrium, and becoming implanted. Most of the cells of the embryo at this stage go into the formation of the placenta. The implanted embryo continues development. HCG stimulates progesterone to replace the secretions of the corpus luteum, and ensure the continued health of the endometrium. Failure at this stage would lead to the loss of the endometrium and embryo in menstrual bleeding, the period. This very early miscarriage will not be detectable to the woman, except as a delayed period, perhaps. At least 40 per cent of embryos entering the uterus fail to implant and die. Many implanted embryos will also fail to develop normally and abort. After 14 days implantation is more secure and the rate of spontaneous abortion (miscarriage) falls, but not, of course, to zero.

Appendix III: Investigation of infertility

The Infertility Clinic conducted by Professor Ian Cooke at the Jessop Hospital for Women, at the time of this study (now much altered), pursued the pattern of investigations described here. It should be noted that this is a generalised description; in many cases results obtained before first attendance or in the earliest tests would lead to advancing some tests or omitting others. The process is in reality individualised. Practical constraints and the availability of both partners also influenced the actual pattern in specific cases.

Normal results in the primary tests on one partner will lead to concentration on the other, with a return to further tests if the problem in one partner is resolved and conception still does not occur. In reality, as with recorded practice at other clinics, it appeared that the woman was more likely to be further investigated, despite satisfactory early results and unsatisfactory ones in the man, than the reverse. This is partly a reflection of the more extensive understanding of female than male infertility. Philipp and Carruthers (1981) advocate baseline investigation of the woman as the starting point without justification of this practice. This and other differences in the treatment of the sexes are discussed in the results.

Visit 1

Physical examination – assessment of reproductive organs
Weight, height and blood pressure   (W only)
Blood and urine test – assessment of hormone levels
                      – check for infections   (W only)
Medical and surgical history – for diseases, events of significance for
      fertility, e.g. injuries, operations, infections
Sexual and obstetric history – for pregnancies, frequency of sexual
      intercourse, sexual practices
Social history – details of habits of relevance, e.g. type of work, alcohol
      and tobacco consumption

BBT instruction – charts to be available at later visit for information on ovulation.

HSG appointment prior to Visit 2.
Semen analysis prior to Visit 2.

Visit 2

Results of tests and treatment instituted for any infections
BBT charts examined for evidence of ovulation
HSG evaluated – patency of tubes
                – structure of uterus
                – presence of obstructions
Semen analysis evaluated.

Thereafter the pattern of visits and tests is tailored to individual needs. This Clinic did not use the post-coital test routinely as used in many clinics on the grounds that it does not usually offer much additional evidence or conclusive results that are not obtainable by other means; it is also a distressing test. Similarly, AIH was not offered, on the grounds that it was more appropriate to treat the hostility factor or sexual problem than use a short cut. It was regarded as having proven value only in cases of a sperm-delivery problem such as retrograde ejaculation.

The main investigations and treatments would be as follows. It should be remembered that the period of this study was one of unprecedented development in the treatment of infertility, and new procedures were being introduced, some of which did not affect all the couples I studied, and some of which were abandoned as having not achieved demonstrable efficacy.

Woman

laparoscopy
antibiotic treatment of infections
hormonal treatment for ovulation
surgical treatment of congenital anomalies, adhesions, PCO, fibroids
    or polyps
drug treatment of endometriosis
microsurgery of tubal obstruction
hormone pump therapy
DI
IVF

Man

repeat semen analyses
testicular biopsy
antibiotic treatment of infections
hormonal treatment of poor semen or immunological problems
surgical treatment of varicocele, congenital anomalies or tubal obstruction
DI
IVF

Appendix IV: Fertility problems
Summary of problems, causes and treatments

This account is highly summarised; detailed discussion may be found in Stangel (1979), Stanway (1984) and Winston (1986 and 1990) which are the principal sources for this summary, as well as the advice of Professor Cooke. Substantial controversy surrounds the significance of some of these problems for fertility, and the efficacy of some treatments. This summary cannot be regarded as conclusive. Not all of the procedures mentioned were in use at the Clinic at the time of the research, and some are no longer in use there. They may, however, be encountered in other descriptions of infertility practice.

INADEQUATE SEMEN ANALYSIS/DEPOSITION

Assessment of sperm quality is primarily by microscopic assessment of semen sample, supported by post-coital test, vasogram (X-ray of reproductive tract), hormonal assay and testicular biopsy. Only first and last were routinely used at this Clinic at the time. Recent innovations include zona-free hamster egg penetration test, ATP concentration, swim-up and velocity tests and IVF.

The definition of 'adequate' is a matter of uncertainty. Barratt *et al.* (1990) suggest a volume in excess of 0.5 ml, at least 20 million sperm per ml semen, 50 per cent motile and 30 per cent or more able to progress, 50 per cent with normal morphology. They do conclude, however, that 'semen parameters are very poor predictors of fertility'.

Assessment of the adequacy of semen deposition will depend on the couple's account of coital practice and physical examination. Semen must be deposited in the vagina near enough to the cervix to enable the sperm to proceed onwards. Poor motility will increase the importance of the semen being deposited at the most effective site, high in the vagina.

1. *Low sperm count*

Condition	Treatment
overweight	diet
excessive exercise	moderate exercise
drugs (e.g. antihypertensives, antidepressants, alcohol, tobacco)	exclude some, reduce others
testes too hot (e.g. sitting for long periods, exposure to heat, constricting clothing)	appropriate advice
varicocele (varicose vein in scrotum)	surgery in severe cases
hormonal problems – lowered testosterone	replacement therapy
– raised LH or FSH	untreatable
– lowered LH or FSH	replacement therapy (value doubted at this Clinic)
– raised prolactin (controversial)	surgery of pituitary tumour; bromocriptine; (empirical treatment with mesterolone)
immunological problems	steroids to suppress antibodies (value doubted)

2. *Poor sperm motility*

testicular failure	generally untreatable
inadequacy of maturation	generally untreatable
varicocele (controversial)	surgery

3. *Azoospermia*

retrograde ejaculation	sperm retrieval and AIH
testicular failure	generally untreatable
structural blockage	microsurgery

4. *Abnormal morphology*

as item 2 above	surgery unlikely

5. *Reduced quantity semen*

gland inflammation	antibiotics
structural abnormality	microsurgery

6. *Sperm clumping*

infection	antibiotics
immunological problems	steroid therapy
	semen 'washing'

7. *Semen fails to liquefy*
infection	antibiotics
chemical imbalance	drug treatment

8. *Mucus penetration failure*
probably chemical problem in sperm	generally untreatable

9. *Semen deposition problems*
hypospadias	surgery
	AIH
coital problem	counselling/advice
impotence	counselling/advice
vaginismus	counselling/advice
	AIH
unruptured hymen	counselling advice
constricted vagina	surgery/dilatation

10. *Ovum penetration failure*
	microinsemination

Where there are cervical hostility or immunological problems, the semen fails to liquefy, there is a physical problem or severe oligospermia, the husband's semen may be collected and concentrated and given to the woman, AIH. The benefits of this are controversial, and it is not undertaken at this Clinic.

In cases of untreatable oligospermia or azoospermia, a couple will be offered DI in which donated semen is inserted into the cervix or uterus of the woman. An embryo thus formed is the biological progeny of the mother and donor. (Semen is now stored and frozen for at least six months since the advent of AIDS, to ensure the identification of possibly dormant human immuno-deficiency virus (HIV), the causative agent of AIDS.)

Ovulatory problems

Ovulation is inferred from the BBT chart and by checking the cervical mucus and hormonal assay. Confirmation is sought through direct visualisation of the ovaries by laparoscopy around the anticipated time of ovulation, endometrial biopsy shortly before a period is due, ovarian biopsy or ultrasound scanning.

This is the area of fertility problems with which there is the most success; Winston suggests a 90 per cent chance of starting ovulation.

1. *Failure of ovulation*

Condition	Treatment
hormonal problem	clomiphene citrate (Clomid)
– lowered FSH and LH	HMG (Pergonal)
	pump therapy with GnRH
– failure of LH surge	HCG after HMG, FSH, or clomiphene
– raised prolactin	bromocriptine
– lowered progesterone	progesterone or retroprogesterone
follicle problem	
– failure of LH surge	HCG

2. *Polycystic ovarian disease (PCO)*

wedge resection (removing small wedge of the ovary)
clomiphene, HMG or FSH

3. *Ovarian failure*

untreatable

4. *Ovarian abnormality*
congenital, iatrogenic or traumatic   untreatable

Tubal problems and endometriosis

The first test done to assess the patency of the fallopian tubes is the HSG, in which radio opaque dye is injected through the tubes via the cervix under X-ray. The course of the dye is observed to see if it spills freely from the fimbrial end of both of the tubes. In addition, the dye will demonstrate the site and nature of any obstruction to the flow, which cannot otherwise be seen as the tubes are so fine. This procedure is frequently repeated at laparoscopy so that the spill, and in some cases the obstruction, may be directly observed.

Blockage or narrowing of the tubes may be partial or, less frequently, complete. There may be damage to the lining of the tubes or the muscle wall, or adhesions developing at the site of damage or scarring which prevent the free movement of the tubes.

Endometriosis is little understood. Unless it is so severe as to obstruct the tubes, which is rare, the relevance of this condition to infertility is controversial. (A recent study at this Clinic suggested that treatment made no difference to fertility.) The practice at this Clinic was the general one of treating it unless it is very mild or causing no symptoms, e.g. heavy or irregular periods, painful intercourse. It is now believed that treatment is unlikely to improve fertility. Being the growth of endometrium albeit away from the normal site in the uterus, this responds to the same hormones as cause the sloughing of the endometrium at menstruation, and is 'cured' by the menopause or pregnancy. Hormone treatments mimic these natural 'remedies'. Pregnancy cannot occur during treatment.

1. *Blockage or obstruction of the tube*

Condition	Treatment
infections, previous pregnancy (particularly ectopic), IUD, pelvic inflammatory disease, congenital abnormalities	tubal insufflation salpingostomy microsurgical anastomosis

2. *Adhesions*

previous surgery, scarring through disease or injury	salpingolysis microsurgery at laparoscopy or open operation

3. *Endometriosis*

cause unknown	contraceptive pill hormone treatment – progesterone – Danazol (synthetic testosterone)

Severe cases of impairment of the tubes are the principal reasons for *in-vitro* fertilisation, which enables fertilisation of the egg and return to the uterus for implantation and development. The little known action of the tube itself in the very early stages of development may account for the high failure rate of this treatment, at least 70 per cent with three embryos, 92 per cent with one (Winston 1986). The new technique of GIFT, where there is some patent and viable tube at the proximal (uterus) end, is intended to overcome this problem.

Uterine problems

These problems are less common than others, and more likely to be overlooked. They would be identified by physical examination, HSG, D&C, ultrasound, hysteroscopy or laparoscopy. The problems connected with fibroids, polyps, adhesions and deformations of the uterus are usually supposed to be physical obstruction of the process of implantation, or possibly of the sperm as they swim up towards the tubes. Adenomyosis is the name for endometriosis when it occurs in the uterine wall.

1. *Fibroids*
   | Condition | Treatment |
   | benign tumour, cause unknown | myomectomy |

2. *Polyps*
   | small growth like fibroid, cause uncertain | curettage |

3. *Adhesions*
   | at site of scarring caused by pregnancy, infections or surgery | surgical division |

4. *Inflammation of uterine lining*
   | infection | antibiotics |
   | IUD, foreign body | removal |

5. *Congenital deformation*
   | partial or complete division of uterus | surgery in severe cases |
   | retroverted uterus (controversial) | not treated |

6. *Adenomyosis*
   | cause uncertain | treatment like endometriosis |

The treatment of these problems is fairly straightforward and successful in many cases. The advent of the hysteroscope and laparoscope has made many of these procedures much less complex, eliminating the need for major surgery. Microsurgery is to be preferred given the dangers ordinary surgery raises of scarring, infections and adhesions.

Cervical problems

Difficulties may arise in this area with the structure of the cervix itself and also with the mucus secreted there which has important functions in the exclusion of infection from the reproductive tract and the control of entry of the sperm.

The matter of mucus problems is perhaps the most controversial in infertility investigation. According to Winston, some doctors regard these 'problems' as fantasy, others as the single most important area of concern. He estimates they affect some 5 per cent of infertile women. Structural problems are identified by physical examination. Mucus tests are the PCT and ferning test. At this Clinic the PCT was little used as discussed in relation to semen problems.

1. *Narrowed or scarred cervix*

Condition	Treatment
injury, difficult childbirth, abortion	dilatation laser or cryogenic (freezing) treatment

2. *Immunological factor in mucus (mucus hostility)*

antibodies to sperm	temporary abstinence from intercourse, or use of condom to permit natural disappearance of antibodies AIH into uterus steroids test fertilisation and IVF

3. *Mucus traps sperm*

poor sperm	(see above)
thick mucus	oestrogen treatment ultrasound assessment of follicle growth
failure of ovulation	(see above)
infected cervix	antibiotics

4. *Inadequate mucus*

ovulation problem	(see above)
hormonal deficit	oestrogen treatment
side effect of ovulatory treatments, e.g. clomiphene, tamoxifen	adjust dosage and/or timing oestrogen treatment

These difficulties can often be successfully treated. IVF may be the only solution; antibodies may also prevent fertilisation outside the body necessitating DI.

Unexplained infertility

This is clearly the residual category used when no cause has been identified for continued failure to conceive. Misleadingly, it is used sometimes as if it were a diagnosis. Criticism of this may be seen in Lenton *et al.* (1977) and Winston (1990). Reference was made in the text to the way it has been used to justify claims for the psychogenesis of infertility (see Chapter 3).

Winston notes that imperfect medical knowledge will be a factor, but also, he claims, failure to conduct all necessary tests to the highest level of detail and care. This may be related to factors of both economics and expertise. Winston (1986: 160) notes the following common omissions during investigation:

– adequate X-rays of tubes and uterus
– hysteroscopy
– carefully timed PCT
– repeated semen analysis
– most recent sperm tests – swim-up and velocity
– thorough hormone tests of male and female
– ultrasound scanning of ovaries to assess follicle development and to check for PCO.

N.B. The glossary gives explanations of the terms used in this summary.

Bibliography

ABAFA (1977) *Child Adoption*, London: Association of British Adoption and Fostering Agencies.

Abse, D.W. (1966) 'Psychiatric aspects of human male infertility', *Fertility and Sterility* 17: 133–9.

Adam, I. (1969) *George Eliot*, London: Routledge & Kegan Paul.

Albee, E. (1962) *Who's Afraid of Virginia Woolf?*, London: Penguin.

Aldgate, J. (1982) 'Foster and adoptive families', in R.N. Rapoport, M.P. Fogarty and R. Rapoport *Families in Britain*, London: Routledge and Kegan Paul.

Amuzu, B., Laxova, R. and Shapiro, S.S. (1990) 'Pregnancy outcome, health of children and family adjustment after donor insemination', *Obstetric Gynecology* 75, 6: 899–905.

Anderson, I. (1985) 'How IUD's cause infertility', *New Scientist* 6: 18/4/85.

Anderson, M. (ed.) (1971) *Sociology of the Family*, England: Penguin.

Arber, S. and Sawyer, L. (1985) 'The role of the receptionist in general practice: a "dragon behind the desk"?', *Social Science and Medicine* 20, 9: 911–21.

Archbishop of Canterbury (1948) Report of a Commission appointed by His Grace the Archbishop of Canterbury, *Artificial Human Insemination*, London: SPCK.

The Archers (1989) Radio 4 Series, London: British Broadcasting Corporation.

Arditti, R. and Duelli Klein, R. (1984) *Test Tube Women: What Future for Motherhood?* London: Routledge & Kegan Paul.

BAAF (1984) *Adopting a Child: A Brief Guide for Prospective Adopters*, London: British Agencies for Adoption and Fostering.

Balchin, N. (1945) *Mine Own Executioner*, London: Collins.

—— (1951) *A Way Through the Wood*, London: Collins.

Bancroft, J. (1983) *Human Sexuality and its Problems*, Edinburgh: Churchill Livingstone.

Barratt, C.L.R., Chauhan, M. and Cooke, I.D. (1990) 'Donor insemination – a look to the future', *Fertility and Sterility* 54, 3: 375–87.

Barry, M.J. (1961) 'Emotional transactions in the pre-adoptive study', in R.Tod, op. cit.

Baum, F.E. (1980) 'Childless by choice: a sociological study of a demographic phenomenon in Britain', unpublished PhD thesis, University of Nottingham.

—— (1982) 'Voluntary childlessness and contraception: problems and practice', *Journal of Biosocial Science* 14: 17–23.

Baum, F. and Cope, D.R. (1980) 'Some characteristics of intentionally childless wives in Britain', *Journal of Biosocial Science* 12: 287–99.

Bazin, G. (1958) *A Concise History of Art*, London: Thames & Hudson.

Becker, G.S. (1960) 'An economic analysis of fertility', in Universities National Bureau for Economic Research, *Demographic and Economic Change in Developed Countries*, Princeton University Press.

Bierkens, P.B. (1975) 'Childlessness from the psychological point of view', *Bulletin of the Menninger Clinic* 39, 2: 177–82.

Binder, P. (1972) *Magic Symbols of the World*, London: Hamlyn.

Black, D. (1980) *The Black Report; Report of the Working Group on Inequalities in Health*, London: DHSS.

Blake, J. (1979) 'Is zero preferred?', *Journal of Marriage and the Family* 41: 245.

Blizzard, J. (1977) *Blizzard and the Holy Ghost*, London: Peter Owen.

Blood, R.O. and Wolfe, D.M. (1955) *Husbands and Wives*, Chicago: Free Press.

Boulton, M.G. (1983) *On Being a Mother: A Study of Women with Pre-School Children*, London: Tavistock.

Bowlby, J. (1965) *Child Care and the Growth of Love*, London: Penguin.

—— (1969) *Attachment and Loss*, London: Hogarth.

Branfoot, G. (1983) *The Wife Wants a Child*, London: Methuen.

Brannen, J. and Collard, J. (1982) *Marriages in Trouble*, London: Tavistock.

Brearley, M. (1986) 'Counsellors and clients: men or women', *Marriage Guidance* 22: 3–9.

Brecher, R. and Brecher, E. (eds) (1966) *An Analysis of Human Sexual Response*, Toronto: New American Library.

BBC (1986) *Bodymatters*, television series, London: British Broadcasting Corporation.

Broome, A. and Wallace, L. (1984) *Psychology and Gynaecological Problems*, London: Tavistock.

Brown, G.W. and Harris, T. (1978) *The Social Origins of Depression: A Study of Psychiatric Disorder in Women*, London: Tavistock.

Burgoyne, J. (1987) 'Change, gender and the life course', in G. Cohen *Social Change and the Life Course*, London: Tavistock.

Burslem, R.W. and Osborn, J.C. (1986) 'Unexplained infertility', *British Medical Journal* 292: 576–7.

Busfield, J. (1974) 'Ideologies and reproduction', in M.P.M. Richards *The Integration of the Child into a Social World*, Cambridge: Cambridge University Press.

Busfield, J. and Paddon, M. (1977) *Thinking about Children: Sociology and Fertility in Post-war England*, London: Cambridge University Press.

Butrym, Z. and Horder, J. (1983) *Health, Doctors and Social Workers*, London: Routledge & Kegan Paul.

Campbell, E. (1975) 'The American way of mating', *Psychology Today* May: 37–43.

—— (1985) *The Childless Marriage: an Exploratory Study of Couples Who Do Not Want Children*, London: Tavistock.

Caplan, G. (1961) *An Approach to Community Mental Health*, London: Tavistock.

Cartwright, A. (1967) *Patients and their Doctors: A Study of General Practice*, London: Routledge & Kegan Paul.

—— (1976) *How Many Children?*, London: Routledge & Kegan Paul.

Cartwright, A. and Anderson, R. (1981) *General Practice Revisited: A Second Study of Patients and their Doctors*, London: Tavistock.

CSO (Central Statistical Office) (1986) *Social Trends No. 16*, London: HMSO.

—— (1989) *Social Trends No. 19*, London: HMSO.

Chertok, L. (1969) *Motherhood and Personality*, London: Tavistock.

Chesler, P. (1974) *Women and Madness*, London: Allen Lane.

Chester, R. (1972) 'Childlessness and marriage breakdown', *Journal of Biosocial Science* 4, 4: 443–54.

CIPFA (1990) *Personal Social Service Statistics: 1988–89 Actuals*, London: Chartered Institute of Public Finance and Accountancy.

Congregation for the Doctrine of the Faith (1987) *Instruction on Respect for Human Life in its Origins and on the Dignity of Procreation: Replies to Certain Questions of the Day*, Rome: Roman Catholic Church.

Connolly, K.J., Edelmann, R.J. and Cooke, I.D. (1987) 'Distress and marital problems associated with infertility', *Journal of Reproductive and Infant Psychology* 5: 49–57.

Cooke, I.D. (1976) 'The natural history and major causes of infertility', paper given at WHO Symposium on Advances in Fertility Regulation, Moscow: World Health Organisation.

Coombe, V. (1976) 'Health and Social Services and Minority Ethnic Groups', *Journal of the Royal Society of Health* 96.

Coombe, V. and Little, A. (1986) *Race and Social Work: A Guide to Training*, London: Tavistock.

Cooper, J.D. (1978) *Patterns of Family Placement – Current Issues in Fostering and Adoption*, London: National Children's Bureau.

Cooper, P.E., Cumber, B. and Hartner, R. (1978) 'Decision making patterns and post-decision adjustment of childfree husbands and wives', *Alternative Lifestyles* 1, 1: 71–94.

Crowe, C. (1987) 'Women want it: in vitro fertilisation and women's motivations for participation', in P. Spallone and D.L. Steinberg (eds) *Made to Order*, London: Pergamon.

Daniluk, J.C., Leader, A. and Taylor, P.J. (1987) 'Psychological and relationship changes of couples undergoing infertility investigations: some implications for counselling', *British Journal of Guidance and Counselling* 15: 29–36.

Davidson, K.W. and Clarke, S.S. (1989) *Social Work in Health Care*, London: Howarth Press.

Dawkins, R. (1976) *The Selfish Gene*, London: Oxford University Press.

Debrovner, C.H. and Shubin-Stein, R. (1976) 'Sexual problems associated with infertility', *Medical Aspects of Human Sexuality* 10: 161–2.

Denber, H.C. (1978) 'Psychiatric aspects of infertility', *Journal of Reproductive Medicine*, 20, 1: 23–9.

Denber, H.C.B. and Roland, M. (1963) 'Psychologic factors and infertility', *Journal of Reproductive Medicine* 2: 285.

Department of Health (1989) *Health and Personal Social Services Statistics for England*, London: HMSO.

—— (1990) *The Nature and Effect of Adoption: Report of the Working Group on Adoption Law in England and Wales*, London: Department of Health.

DHSS (Department of Health & Social Security) (1976) *Guide to Fostering Practice*, London: DHSS.

Deutsch, H. (1945) *The Psychology of Women*, vol. 2, New York: Grune & Stratton.

Diczfalusy, E. (1986) 'WHO special programme of research, development and research training in human reproduction – the first fifteen years: a review', *Contraception* 34: 1.

Dominian, J. (1968) *Marital Breakdown*, London: Penguin.
Dowrick, S. and Grundberg, S. (eds) (1980) *Why Children?*, London: Women's Press.
Dunnell, K. (1979) *Family Formation 1976*, London: HMSO.
Eastenders (1988) BBC 1 television series, London: British Broadcasting Corporation.
Edelmann, R.J. and Connolly, K.J. (1986) 'Psychological aspects of infertility', *British Journal of Medical Psychology* 59: 209–19.
Ehrenreich, B. and English, D. (1974) *Complaints and Disorders – The Sexual Politics of Sickness*, Glass Mountain Pamphlet No.2, London: Compendium.
Eichenbaum, L. and Orbach, S. (1983) *What Do Women Want?*, London: Michael Joseph.
Eisenthal, S. and Lazare, A. (1976) 'Evaluation of the interaction in a walk-in clinic', *Journal of Nervous and Mental Disorders* 162: 169–75.
Eliot, G. (1967) *Silas Marner*, London: Penguin.
Erikson, E. (1950) *Childhood and Society*, London: Penguin.
Eysenck, H.J. (1986) *The Decline and Fall of the Freudian Empire*, London: Penguin.
Farid, S.M. (1974) *Current Tempo of Fertility in England and Wales*, London: HMSO.
Feversham Committee (1960) *Report of the Departmental Committee on Human Artificial Insemination*, Cmnd 1105, London: HMSO.
Firestone, S. (1972) *The Dialectic of Sex*, St Albans: Paladin.
Fischer, J. and Gochros, H.L. (1977) *Handbook of Behavior Therapy with Sexual Problems. Vol.II; Approaches to Specific Problems*, New York: Pergamon.
Fitzpatrick, R. (1984) 'Satisfaction with health care', in R. Fitzpatrick *et al. The Experience of Illness*, London: Tavistock.
Foss, G.L. (1982) 'AID – a review of twelve years' experience', *Journal of the Biosocial Society* 14: 253–62.
Freeman, E.W., Garcia, C.R. and Rickels, K. (1983) 'Behavioural and emotional factors – comparison of anovulatory infertile women with fertile and other infertile women', *Fertility and Sterility* 40: 195–201.
Froggatt, R.C. (1982) 'Why not a sub-fertility co-operation card?' *Journal of the Royal College of General Practitioners* 32: 316.
Froggatt, C. (1983) 'Problems of fertility and their management', *Journal of the Royal College of General Practitioners* 33: 171–4.
Garcia, C.A., Freeman, E.W., Rickels, K., Chung Wu, Scholl, G., Galle, P.C. and Boxer, A.S. (1985) 'Behavioural and emotional factors and treatment responses in a study of anovulatory infertile women', *Fertility and Sterility* 44: 478–85.
Garcia Lorca, F. (1987) 'Yerma', in *Three Tragedies*, London: Methuen.
Garde, K. and Lunde, I. (1980) 'Female sexual behavior. A study in a random sample of 40 year old women', *Maturitas* 2: 225–40.
Gebhard, P.H. and Johnson, A.B. (1979) *The Kinsey Data: Marginal Tabulations of the 1938–1963 Interviews Conducted by the Institute for Sex Research*, Philadelphia: Saunders.
Gibson, C. (1980) 'Childlessness and marital instability: a re-examination of the evidence', *Journal of Biosocial Science* 12, 1: 121–32.
Giele-Zwier, T. (1971) *Onvruchtbaarheid en Huwelijkssatisfactie*, NISSO Report, Institute for Socio-Sexological Research; Netherlands.
Goffman, E. (1961) *Asylums: Essays on the Social Situation of Mental Patients and other Inmates*, London: Penguin.

—— (1963) *Stigma: Notes on the Management of Spoiled Identity*, Englewood Cliffs, NJ: Prentice-Hall.

HFEA (1991) *Code of Practice: Consultation Document*, London: Human Fertilisation and Embryology Authority.

Halbwachs, M. (1930) *The Causes of Suicide*, trans. H. Goldblatt, 1978, London: Routledge & Kegan Paul.

Hanssen, M. (1984) *E for Additives: The Complete E Number Guide*, Wellingborough: Thorsons.

Harper, R., Lenton, E.A. and Cooke, I.D. (1985) 'Prolactin and subjective reports of stress in women attending an infertility clinic', *Journal of Reproductive and Infant Psychology* 3: 3–8.

Hart, N. (1976) *When Marriage Ends: A Study in Status Passage*, London: Tavistock.

Heywood, J.S. (1978) *Children in Care: The Development of the Service for the Deprived Child*, London: Routledge & Kegan Paul.

Hirsch, M.B. and Mosher, W.D. (1987) 'Characteristics of infertile women in the United States and their use of infertility services', *Fertility and Sterility* 47, 4: 618–25.

Hoffman, L.W. and Hoffman, M.L. (1973) 'The value of children to parents', in J. Fawcett (ed.) *Psychological Perspectives on Population*, New York: Basic Books.

Houghton, P. and Houghton, D. (1977) *Unfocussed Grief: Responses to Childlessness*, Birmingham: Birmingham Settlement.

Houghton, D. and Houghton, P. (1984) *Coping with Childlessness*, London: George Allen & Unwin.

Houseknecht, S. (1979) 'The timing of the decision to remain childless. evidence for continuous socialisation', *Psychology of Women Quarterly* 4, 1: 81–96.

Howe, G., Westhoff, C., Vessey, M. and Yeates, D. (1985) 'Effects of age, cigarette smoking and other factors on fertility. Findings in a large prospective study', *British Medical Journal* 290: 1697–1700.

Hull, M.G.R., Glazener, C.M.A., Kelly, N.J., Conway, D.I., Foster, P.A., Hinton, R.A., Coulson, C., Lambert, P.A., Watt, E.M. and Desai, K.M. (1985) 'Population study of the causes, treatment and outcome of infertility', *British Medical Journal* 291: 1693–7.

Humphrey, M. (1969) *The Hostage Seekers: A Study of Childless and Adopting Couples*, London: Longman.

Humphrey, M. and Humphrey, H. (1987) 'Marital relationships in couples seeking donor insemination', *Journal of Biosocial Science* 19, 2: 209–19

Hunt, M. (1974) *Sexual Behavior in the 1970s*, Chicago: Playboy Press.

Hunt, P.A. (1985) *Clients' Responses to Marriage Counselling*, Research Report No.3, National Marriage Guidance Council, Rugby.

ILA (Interim Licensing Authority) (1990) *The Fifth Report of the Interim Licensing Authority for Human In Vitro Fertilisation and Embryology*, London.

Issue (1986–), Journal of the National Association for the Childless, Birmingham: Birmingham Settlement.

JWPT (1991) Personal communication from staff member of the Jersey Wildlife Preservation Trust.

James, W.H. (1986) 'Recent secular trends in dizygotic twinning rates in Europe', *Journal of Biosocial Science* 18: 497–504.

Jequier, A.M. (1986) *Infertility in the Male*, Edinburgh: Churchill Livingstone.

Jones, C.C. (1967) *Social and Psychological Factors in Pregnancy*, Dissertation for the degree of Master of Arts, Liverpool University.

Jones, M. (1991) *Infertility: Modern Treatments and the Issues They Raise*, London: Piatkus.

Kaplan,H.S. (1978) *The New Sex Therapy: Active Treatment of Sexual Dysfunctions*, London: Penguin.

Karahasanoglu, A., Barglow, P. and Growe, G. (1972) 'Psychological aspects of infertility', *Journal of Reproductive Medicine* 9, 5: 241–7.

Keye, W. (1982) 'Avoiding iatrogenic infertility', in *Resolve Newsletter*, April; National Organisation of Non-parents, New York.

Klein, R. (ed.) (1989) *The Exploitation of Infertility: Women and Reproductive Technologies*, London: Women's Press.

Korer, J. & Fitzsimmons, J.S. (1985) 'The effect of Huntingdon's Chorea on family life', *British Journal of Social Work* 15: 581–97.

Kornitzer, M. (1968) *Adoption and Family Life*, London: Putnam.

Ladeira, M. (1977) 'Estudo comparativo e avaliação psicoterapica de pacientes inférteis', *Revista de Ginecologia e d'Obstetrica* 134: 87–94.

Lamson, H.D., Pinard, W.J. and Meaker, S.R. (1951) 'Sociologic and psychological aspects of artificial insemination with donor semen', *Journal of the American Medical Association* 145: 1062–4.

Last, J. (1963) 'The illness iceberg. Completing the clinical picture in general practice', *Lancet* 2: 28–31.

Laurance, J. (1982) 'The moral pressure to have children', *New Society* 5/8/82: 217.

Lenton, E.A., Weston, G.A. and Cooke, I.D. (1977) 'Long term follow-up of the apparently normal couple with a complaint of infertility', *Fertility and Sterility* 28: 913–9.

Lorenz, K. (1963) *On Aggression*, London: McEwan.

McGregor, O.R. (1957) *Divorce in England*, London: Routledge & Kegan Paul.

Macintyre, S. (1976) 'Who wants babies? The social construction of instincts', in D.L. Barker and S. Allen (eds) *Sexual Divisions and Society. Process and Change*, London: Tavistock.

McLoughlin, J. (1984) 'The case for the conscientious objector to motherhood', *The Guardian* 13/3/84.

Mahlstedt, P. (1985) 'The psychological component of infertility', *Fertility and Sterility* 43, 3: 335–45.

Mai, F.M.M. (1972) 'Psychiatric interview comparisons between infertile and fertile couples', *Psychosomatic Medicine* 34: 431–8.

Mai, F.M.M., Munday, R.N. and Rump, E.E. (1972) 'Psychosomatic and behavioural mechanisms in psychogenic infertility', *British Journal of Psychiatry* 120: 199.

Maitland, S. (1987) *Daughters of Jerusalem*, London: Pan.

Mauksch, H.O. (1972) 'Ideology, patient care and interaction in hospitals', paper presented at the Third International Conference on Social Science and Medicine, Elsinore, Denmark.

Mazor, M.D. and Simons, H.F. (1984) (eds) *Infertility – Medical, Emotional and Social Consequences*, New York: Human Services Press.

Mazure, C.M. and Greenfeld, D.A. (1989) 'Psychological studies of in vitro fertilisation/embryo transfer participants', *Journal of In Vitro Fertilisation and Embryo Transfer* 6, 4: 242–56.

Mead, M. (1949) *Male and Female*, New York: Morrow.

Mead, M. and Newton, N. (1967) 'Cultural patterning of perinatal behaviour', in S.A. Richardson and A.F. Guttsmacher op. cit.

Mechanic, D. and Volkart, E. (1961) 'Stress, illness behaviour and the sick role', *American Sociological Review* 20: 51–8.

Menning, B.E. (1977) *Infertility: A Guide for the Childless Couple*, Englewood Cliffs, NJ: Prentice Hall.

—— (1980) 'The emotional needs of infertile couples', *Fertility and Sterility* 34, 4: 313–19.

Miall, C.E. (1984) 'Women and involuntary childlessness: perceptions of stigma associated with infertility and adoption', unpublished PhD thesis, York University, Toronto, Canada.

—— (1986) 'The stigma of involuntary childlessness', *Social Problems* 33, 4: 268–82.

Monach, J.H. (1985) 'Experiences of the treadmill', *NACK: Journal of the National Association for the Childless*, Summer.

—— (1987) 'An investigation of involuntary childlessness and of the strategies of help offered', unpublished PhD thesis, University of Sheffield.

Moulder, C. (1990) *Miscarriage: Women's Experiences and Needs*, London: Pandora.

NACK: Journal of the National Association for the Childless, 1976–1986, Birmingham: Birmingham Settlement.

NAHA (1987) Poll conducted by Marplan for the National Association of Health Authorities on views of the public concerning the National Health Service. Quoted in *Family Practitioner Services: Journal of the Society of Administrators of Family Practitioner Services*, May.

NAOP (National Alliance for Optional Parenthood) *Questions and Answers: Optional Parenthood Today*, Washington. (Undated leaflet.)

—— (1979) *Pronatalism*, Washington.

Newill, R. (1974) *Infertile Marriage*, London: Penguin.

—— (1981) Letter published in *NACK* op. cit.

Newson, J. and Newson, E.N. (1965) *Patterns of Infant Care in an Urban Community*, London: Penguin.

Norris, A.S. (1965) 'Psychological aspects of infertility', *Journal of Iowa Medical Society* LV, 3: 122–4.

Noy, P., Wollstein, S. and Atara Kaplan-de-Nour (1966) 'Clinical observations on the psychogenesis of impotence', *British Journal of Medical Psychology* 39: 43–53.

O'Brien, M. (1988) 'Men and fathers in therapy', *Journal of Family Therapy* 10: 109–23.

Oakley, A. (1979) *Becoming a Mother*, Oxford: Martin Robertson.

—— (1981) *Subject Women*, Oxford: Martin Robertson.

—— (1984) *The Captured Womb: A History of the Medical Care of Pregnant Women*, Oxford: Basil Blackwell.

OPCS (Office of Population Censuses and Surveys) (1968) *The General Household Survey 1966*, London: HMSO.

—— (1981a) *Census 1981: County Monitor; South Yorkshire*, London: HMSO.

—— (1981b) *Census 1981*, London: HMSO.

—— (1983) *The General Household Survey 1981*, London: HMSO.

—— (1984) *Birth Statistics. Review of the Registrar General on Births and Patterns of Family Building in England and Wales 1981*, Series FM1 No.8, London: HMSO.

—— (1986a) *Adoption Statistics 1984*, London: HMSO.

—— (1986b) *Birth Statistics 1984, Review of the Registrar General on Births and Patterns of Family Building in England and Wales 1981*, London: HMSO.

—— (1986c) *The General Household Survey 1985*, London: HMSO.

—— (1987) *Divorces in England and Wales 1986*, Series FM2 87/2, London: HMSO.

—— (1988) *Abortion Statistics 1987*, Series AB 14, London: HMSO.

—— (1989) *The General Household Survey 1987*, London: HMSO.

—— (1990) *Birth Statistics 1988, Review of the Registrar General on Births and Patterns of Family Building in England and Wales 1985*, London: HMSO.

—— (1991) *Marriage and Divorce Statistics*, Series FM2 No. 17, London: HMSO.

Owens, D. (1979) 'Recourse to the doctor: the definition of involuntary childlessness as a medical problem', paper given at the British Sociological Association, Medical Sociology Group Annual Conference, University of York.

—— (1982) 'The desire to father: reproductive ideologies and involuntarily childless men', in L. McKee and M. O'Brien (eds) *The Father Figure*, London: Tavistock.

—— (1983) 'Study of NAC members views of AID', *NACK: Journal of the National Association for the Childless:* Winter.

Owens, D.J. and Read, M.W. (1979) *The Provision, Use and Evaluation of Medical Services for the Subfertile; An Analysis Based on the Experience of Involuntarily Childless Couples*, Working Paper No.4. Sociological Research Unit, University College, Cardiff.

Pahl, R.E. (1984) *Division of Labour*, Oxford: Basil Blackwell.

Palti, Z. (1969) 'Psychogenic male infertility', *Psychosomatic Medicine*, 31: 326–30.

Parkes, A.S. (1985) *Off-Beat Biologist: An Autobiography*, Cambridge: Galton Foundation.

Parkes, C. Murray (1986) *Bereavement: Studies of Grief in Adult Life*, 2nd edn, London: Tavistock.

Payne, J. (1978) 'Talking about children', *Journal of Biosocial Science* 10: 367–74.

Peck, E. and Senderowitz, E. (eds) (1974) *Pronatalism: The Myth of Mom and Apple Pie*, New York: Crowell.

Peel, J. and Carr, G. (1975) *Contraception and Family Design: A Study of Birth Planning in Contemporary Society*, London: Churchill Livingstone.

Pepperell, R.J. and McBain, J.C. (1985) 'Unexplained infertility: a review', *British Journal of Obstetrics and Gynaecology* 92: 569–80.

Pfeffer, N. and Woollett, A. (1983) *The Experience of Infertility*, London: Virago.

Pfeffer, N. and Quick, A. (1988) *Infertility Services: A Desperate Case*, London: Greater London Association of Community Health Councils.

Philipp, E.E. and Carruthers, G.B. (eds) (1981) *Infertility*, London: Heinemann.

Plath, S. (1981) *Collected Poems*, London: Faber & Faber.

Pohlman, E. (1968) 'Burgess and Cottrell Data on "Desire for Children": an example of distortion in marriage and family textbooks', *Journal of Marriage and the Family* 30, 3: 433–36.

—— (1969) *The Psychology of Birth Planning*, Cambridge, Mass.: Schenkman.

Porter, M. (1980) 'Willing deviants: a study of childlessness', unpublished PhD thesis, University of Aberdeen.

Poster, M. (1978) *Critical Theory of the Family*, London: Pluto Press.

Probst, C. (1982) 'Religion and infertility: feelings from an infertile Mormon', *Resolve Newsletter*, February.

Putnam, S.M., Stiles, W. and Wolf, M. (1979) 'Interaction exchange structure and patient satisfaction with the medical interview', *Medical Care* 17: 667–81.

Qureshi, H. and Walker, A. (1989) *The Caring Relationship: Elderly People and their Families*, Basingstoke: Macmillan.

Rachootin, P. and Olsen, J. (1981) 'Social selection in seeking medical care for reduced fecundity among women in Denmark', *Journal of Epidemiology and Community Health* 35: 262–4.

Rajkumar, R. (1982) 'Social pressures to have children in the Third World', reprinted in *BON Newsletter*.

Raphael-Leff, J. (1990) *The Psychological Processes of Childbearing*, London: Chapman & Hall.

Reeder, S., Marcus, A. and Seeman, T. (1978) 'The influence of social networks on the use of health services', quoted in R. Fitzpatrick *et al.*, *The Experience of Illness*, London: Tavistock.

Reid, J. (1981) Letter in *Social Work Today* 12: 32, 14/4/81.

Reisz, M.J. (1987) 'Choosing childlessness', *New Society* 20–1, 19/6/87.

Rich, A. (1977) *Of Woman Born*, London: Virago.

Richards, M.P.M. (1982) 'How should we approach the study of fathers?', in L. McKee and M. O'Brien (eds) *The Father Figure*, London: Tavistock.

Richardson, S.A. and Guttsmacher, A.F. (1967) *Childbearing – its Social and Psychological Aspects*, New York: Williams & Wilkins.

Robertson, J. (1953) 'Some responses of young children to loss of maternal care', *Nursing Times* 49: 382.

Robinson, R. (1982) *Childs Play*, unpublished play performed in the Crucible Theatre, Sheffield and on Radio 4, British Broadcasting Corporation.

Rocker, I. (1963) 'The value of an infertility clinic', unpublished MD thesis, University of London.

Rollins, B.C. and Cannon, K.L. (1974) 'Marital satisfaction over the family life cycle: a re-evaluation', *Journal of Marriage and the Family* 36, 2: 271–82.

Rowe, J. (1966) *Parents, Children and Adoption: A Handbook for Adoption Workers*, London: Routledge & Kegan Paul.

—— (1969) *Yours by Choice: A Guide for Adoptive Parents*, London: Routledge & Kegan Paul.

Rowe, J. and Lambert, L. (1973) *Children Who Wait; A Study of Children Needing Substitute Families*, London: Association of British Adoption Agencies.

Rudkin, D. (1978) *Ashes*, London: Pluto Press.

Ryan, T. (1985) 'Roots of masculinity', in A. Metcalfe and M. Humphries (eds) *The Sexuality of Men*, London: Pluto Press.

Sand, K. (1935) Die Physiologie des Hodens, Leipzig.

Sanderson, D. (1985) 'Adopters are people, too', *Social Work Today* 11/2/85.

Sandler, B. (1965) 'Conception after adoption; a comparison of conception rates', *Fertility and Sterility* 16: 313–22.

Sawbridge, P. (1980) 'Seeking new parents: a decade of development', in J. Triseliotis (ed.) *New Developments in Foster Care and Adoption*, London: Routledge & Kegan Paul.

Scambler, G. and Scambler, A. (1984) 'The illness iceberg and aspects of consulting behaviour', in R. Fitzpatrick *et al.*, *The Experience of Illness*, London: Tavistock.

Schwartz, M., Jewelewicz, R. and Vande Wiele, R.L. (1980) 'Application of Orthodox Jewish law to reproductive medicine', *Fertility and Sterility* 33, 5: 471–4.

Seastrunk, J.W. (1984) 'Psychological evaluation of couples in an in-patient reproductive biology unit', *Fertility and Sterility* 41, 2 Abstracts Supplement.

Shapiro, C.H. (1988) *Infertility and Pregnancy Loss: A Guide for Helping Professionals*, San Francisco: Jossey Bass.

Shedlin, M. and Hollerbach, P. (1978) *Modern and Traditional Fertility Regulation in a Mexican Community: Factors in the Process of Decision Making*, New York: Center for Policy Studies.

Siemiaticki, J., Campbell, S., Richardson, L. and Aubert, D. (1984) 'Quality of response in different population groups in mail and telephone surveys', *American Journal of Epidemiology* 120, 2: 302–14.

Smale, G.G. (1977) *Prophecy, Behaviour and Change*, London: Routledge & Kegan Paul.

Smith, C.R. (1984) *Adoption and Fostering; Why and How*, London: Macmillan.

Smith, M. (1981) 'Religion and infertility', *Resolve Newsletter*, December.

Snowden, R., Mitchell, G.D. and Snowden, E.M. (1983) *Artificial Reproduction: A Social Investigation*, London: George Allen & Unwin.

Snowden, R. and Mitchell, G.D. (1981) *The Artificial Family: A Consideration of Artificial Insemination by Donor*, London: George Allen & Unwin.

Spallone, P. (1989) *Beyond Conception: The New Politics of Reproduction*, London: Macmillan.

Stangel, J.J. (1979) *Fertility and Conception: An Essential Guide for Childless Couples*, New York: Paddington Press.

Stanway, A. (1980) *Why Us? A Common Sense Guide for the Childless*, London: Granada.

—— (1981) *Overcoming Depression*, London: Hamlyn.

—— (1984) *Infertility: A Common Sense Guide for the Childless*, Wellingborough: Thorsons.

Stanworth, M. (1987) *Reproductive Technologies: Gender, Motherhood and Medicine*, Oxford: Basil Blackwell.

Stengel, E. (1964) *Suicide and Attempted Suicide*, London: Penguin.

Stimson, G. and Webb, B. (1975) *Going to See the Doctor: The Consultation Process in General Practice*, London: Routledge & Kegan Paul.

Storr, A. (1964) *Sexual Deviation*, London: Penguin.

Sutherland, A.T. (1981) *Disabled We Stand*, London: Souvenir.

Taylor, W.J.C. (1982) 'Infertility investigations. A study of the effects of group counselling on mood change and social functioning', unpublished MPhil thesis, University of Edinburgh.

Thomas, A.K. and Forrest, M.S. (1980) 'Infertility; a review of 291 infertile couples over 8 years', *Fertility and Sterility* 34, 2: 106–11.

Thomas, K.B. (1978) 'The consultation and the therapeutic illusion', *British Medical Journal* 1978, 1: 1327–8.

Thornes, B. and Collard, J. (1979) *Who Divorces?*, London: Routledge & Kegan Paul.

Timms, N. and Blampied, A. (1985) *Intervention in Marriage. The Experience of Counsellors and their Clients*, Joint Unit for Social Services Research, University of Sheffield.

Tod, R. (ed.) (1971) *Social Work in Adoption: Collected Papers*, London: Longman.

Townsend, P. (1964) *The Last Refuge*, London: Routledge & Kegan Paul.

Townsend, P. and Davidson, N. (1982) *Inequalities in Health: The Black Report*, London: Penguin.

Treadway, J. (1983) 'Patient satisfaction and the content of GP consultations', *Journal of the Royal College of General Practitiners* 33: 769–71.

Triseliotis, J. (ed.) (1980) *New Developments in Foster Care and Adoption*, London: Routledge & Kegan Paul.

United Nations (1976) *Fertility and Family Planning in Europe around 1970: A Comparative Study of 12 National Surveys*, New York: United Nations.

Valentine, D. (ed.) (1988) *Infertility and Adoption: A Guide for Social Work Practice*, New York: Haworth Press.

Veevers, J.E. (1972) 'The violation of fertility mores: voluntary childlessness as deviant behaviour', in C. Boydell *et al.*, *Deviant Behaviour and Societal Reaction*, Toronto: Holt, Rinehart & Winston.

—— (1979) 'Voluntary childlessness: a review of issues and evidence', *Marriage & Family Review* 2, 2: 1–26.

—— (1980) *Childless by Choice*, Toronto: Butterworth.

Vessey, M.P., Smith, M.A. and Yeates, D. (1986) 'Return of fertility after discontinuation of oral contraceptives. Influence of age and parity', *British Journal of Family Planning* 11: 120–4.

Voysey, M. (1975) *A Constant Burden: the Reconstitution of Family Life*, London: Routledge & Kegan Paul.

Walker, H.E. (1978) 'Psychiatric aspects of infertility', *Urologic Clinics of North America* 5, 3, October: 481–8.

Warnock Report (1984) *Report of the Committee of Inquiry into Human Fertilisation and Embryology*; Chairman, Dame Mary Warnock, Cmnd 9314, London: HMSO.

Welburn, V. (1980) *Postnatal Depression*, London: Fontana.

Wilson, A. (1981) *Black People and the Health Service*, London: Brent Community Health Council.

Wing, J.K. and Brown, G.W. (1970) *Institutionalism and Schizophrenia*, London: Cambridge University Press.

Winnicott, D.W. (1965) *Family and Individual Development*, London: Hogarth Press.

Winston, R.M.L. (1986) *Infertility. A Sympathetic Approach*, London: Martin Dunitz.

—— (1990) *Getting Pregnant*, London: Anaya.

Woolf, M. (1971) *Family Intentions*, London: HMSO.

Wordsworth, W. (1984) *Collected Poems*, Oxford: Oxford University Press.

Wren, B.G. (ed.) (1985) *Handbook of Obstetrics and Gynaegology*, 2nd edn, London: Chapman Hall.

Young, M. and Wilmott, P. (1957) *Family and Kinship in East London*, London: Routledge & Kegan Paul.

Young, M. and Wilmott, P. (1973) *The Symmetrical Family. A Study of Work and Leisure in the London Region*, London: Routledge & Kegan Paul.

Yourti, E., Inui, T.S. and Williamson, J. (1976) 'Improved outcomes in hypertension after physician tutorials: a controlled trial', *Annals of International Medicine* 84: 646–51.

Zola, I.K. (1973) 'Pathways to the doctor: from person to patient', *Social Science and Medicine* 7, 9: 677–89.

Name index

Subject index